BACH
FLOWERS
for
Crisis Care

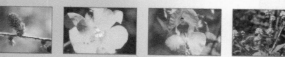

OTHER BOOKS BY MECHTHILD SCHEFFER

Bach Flower Therapy: Theory and Practice

The Encyclopedia of Bach Flower Therapy

Keys to the Soul: A Workbook for Self-Diagnosis Using the Bach Flowers

Mastering Bach Flower Therapies: A Guide to Diagnosis and Treatment

BACH
FLOWERS
for
Crisis Care

Remedies for Emotional
and Psychological Well-being

MECHTHILD SCHEFFER
Translated by Ariel Godwin

Healing Arts Press
Rochester, Vermont • Toronto, Canada

Healing Arts Press
One Park Street
Rochester, Vermont 05767
www.HealingArtsPress.com

Healing Arts Press is a division of Inner Traditions International

Originally published in German under the title *Bach-Blüten-Selbsthilfe in Krisensituationen*
by Heinrich Hugendubel Verlag
First U.S. edition published in 2009 by Healing Arts Press

Note to the reader: This book is intended as an informational guide. The remedies, approaches, and techniques described herein are meant to supplement, and not to be a substitute for, professional medical care or treatment. They should not be used to treat a serious ailment without prior consultation with a qualified health care professional.

Library of Congress Cataloging-in-Publication Data
Scheffer, Mechthild.
 [Bach-Blüten-Selbsthilfe in Krisensituationen. English]
 Bach flowers for crisis care : remedies for emotional and psychological well-being / Mechthild Scheffer ; translated by Ariel Godwin.
  p. cm.
 ISBN 978-1-59477-296-2 (pbk.)
 1. Flowers—Therapeutic use. 2. Homeopathy—Materia medica and therapeutics. 3. Stress (Psychology)—Homeopathic treatment. I. Title.
 RX615.F55S33813 2009
 615.5'32—dc22

                                                          2009006707

Printed and bound in the United States

10 9 8 7 6 5 4 3 2

Text design and layout by Virginia Scott Bowman
This book was typeset in Life with Baskerville and Agenda as display typefaces

Contents

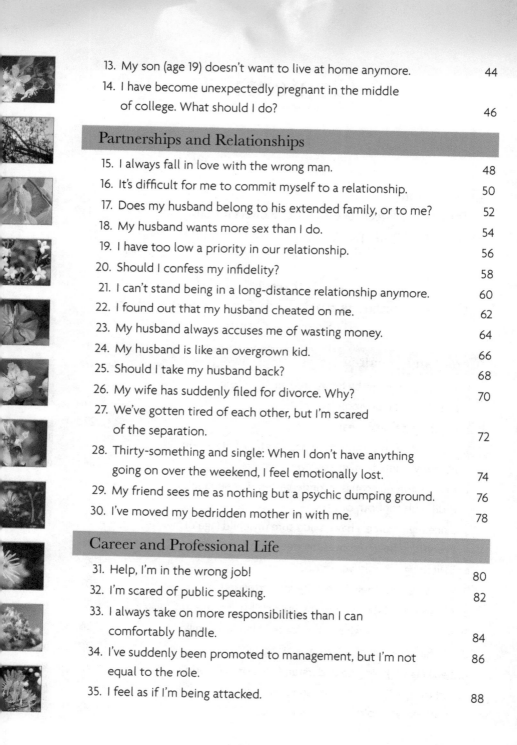

❧ Part 2
The Practical Application of
Bach Flower Therapy

How to Prepare Bach Flower Combinations

The 38 Individual Bach Flower Remedies, Plus Rescue Remedy

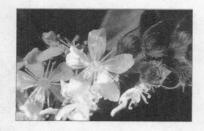

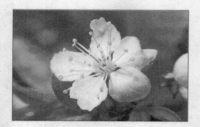

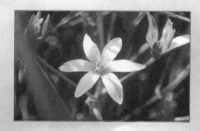

"Crises in themselves are positive. One must simply remove the taste of catastrophe that goes with them."

MAX FRISCH

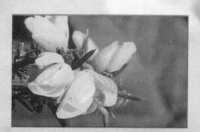

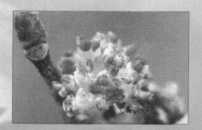

Introduction

The Amazing Effectiveness
of Bach Flowers for Crisis Care

As the saying goes, "The only constant in life is change." *Panta rei*—everything flows—thus the ancient Greeks formulated this important spiritual law. Life is an eternal process of evolution. Those who accept this and go with the flow will have an easier time traveling the river of life. If one blocks this flow, if one struggles against it consciously or unconsciously, then the energy of evolutionary development is blocked. A crisis occurs.

CRISES AS CATALYSTS

A crisis creates the chaos necessary for new movement to take place. The energy of regeneration comes back into flow, enabling the next step in the journey of life. Thus every crisis is an opportunity for psychic self-help.

It does not matter whether a crisis begins as inner discontent, restlessness, helplessness, or an external blow from fate. In keeping with the law "As within, so without," our external crises often reflect our inner spiritual condition.

Crises may strike us out of a clear blue sky, or may fester for years. A crisis always comes—spiritually speaking—at the *right* moment. That is, at the moment in life when the stars have aligned to demand change. In the painful days when a crisis is unfolding, it is often difficult to recognize this.

1

Normally, in crisis situations, we first mobilize our powers of resistance, endeavoring unconsciously to hang on to the status quo. We're anxious and in pain. But at some point, inevitably, the next phase begins: through one or several revealing experiences, we recognize that things cannot continue in the same way, and we then become internally ready to accept change. We become creative—we ponder; we find a better solution; we change our behavior patterns.

But unfortunately, crises can also take a different direction. When the revealing experience is not perceived, or is ignored, life often presents the next opportunity for change in the form of a more intense crisis. Crises cannot be prevented, but one can make the best of them—or the worst.

"Oh, God! I did everything wrong!" people in crisis situations tend to say. This is never correct, because initially a positive outcome is always desired. However, due to lack of awareness or to all-pervasive, destructive beliefs, we sometimes choose the wrong response. It's wrong from the perspective of Bach Flower Therapy, because one has not acted in harmony with spiritual principles.

THE SPIRITUAL CONCEPT OF
THE ORIGINAL BACH FLOWER THERAPY

The original Bach Flower Therapy was developed by English physician and philosopher Edward Bach (1886–1936). Since 1981, Mechthild Scheffer has worked systematically to develop this therapy further.

Bach Flower Therapy is based on the idea that every crisis or physical illness originates from a disturbance of the equilibrium due to a "spiritual misunderstanding" (that is, a misunderstanding of cosmic laws), which manifests in the form of negative or distorted psychic behavior patterns, such as self-punishment, overassertiveness, or indecision. These negative or distorted behavior patterns form "psychic poisons" (psychotoxins) and block access to one's intuitive inner wisdom, which Bach called "Inner Guidance."

Edward Bach discovered and defined "thirty-eight disharmonic psychic conditions of human nature." These thirty-eight states form a repertoire of behavior that can be observed in all people, irrespective of time, race, or culture. Manifesting as symptoms (both emotional and physical), they show us in what areas we've lost our connection to our Inner Guidance and have cut ourselves off from the energy flow.

For each of these thirty-eight distorted psychic states, Bach identified a Flower Essence that would harmonize the negative energies, bringing them back into line with the wisdom of Inner Guidance. The goal of Bach Flower Therapy is to reestablish the psychic equilibrium by equalizing these destructive psychic behavior patterns (for example, self-reproach is reshaped step-by-step into self-respect). When one recognizes the spiritual misunderstanding at the root of a crisis situation, it becomes possible to maneuver out of this psychic cul-de-sac by correcting the misunderstanding. Thus connection with one's Inner Guidance is reestablished, and the way is cleared for personal psychic self-healing. Self-development and psychic growth can once again take place.

THE BACH FLOWER CONCENTRATES

The Bach Flower Concentrates are thirty-eight Flower extracts prepared in a similar manner to homeopathic medicines. Made from wild plants and trees, they form the ingredients of individually prepared Bach Flower Remedies.

Bach called the plants he chose the "happy fellows of the plant world." They intentionally do not include any nutritional or conventional medicinal plants, and their Flowers contain no toxins.

Folk medicine since time immemorial has ascribed certain symbolic qualities to these plants; for example, the oak tree is viewed worldwide as a symbol of strength and endurance.

How They Are Used

A distinction is made among three levels of application.

- **Preventive psychic health.** For developing awareness, strengthening character, and harmonizing dissonant mental behavior patterns, like jealousy, anxiety, and apathy.
- **Emergency treatment for psychic stress situations and life crises.** For example, relationship conflicts, child-development and school problems, work issues, and midlife crises. May be supplemental to psychotherapy.
- **Supplemental treatment for acute and chronic illnesses.** Used in addition to specific treatment by physicians or other healing practitioners.

KEY WORDS FOR THE LIFE PLAN
MODEL OF BACH FLOWER THERAPY

The Soul or Higher Self

In keeping with the great healing traditions of all peoples (such as Ayurveda and Paracelsian medicine), Bach Flower Therapy assumes that in every person there is an immortal, divine part (the Soul, the Higher Self) and a transient part (the personality). This Higher Self endeavors to realize an idea or to develop a "divine" quality (for example, harmony). It designs our Life Purpose and our Life Plan (for example, the steps to becoming a professional musician or licensed psychologist).

Personality and Life Plan

The personality is the human being—the flesh and blood. With the personality as its instrument, the Soul is able to realize its life course. For this purpose, the personality is endowed with specific potential characteristics and gifts (such as perseverance). Via the free and individual development of these positive potential characteristics, the Life Plan can be put into action, step-by-step.

Inner Guidance/Inner Voice

Inner Guidance, as the language of the Higher Self, is the mediator and energetic connection between Soul and personality. Through inspiration and based on spiritual principles, it leads the personality in the gradual unfolding of his or her Life Plan.

THE SPIRITUAL PRINCIPLES OF BACH FLOWER THERAPY

In the spiritual system upon which Bach Flower Therapy is based, two main principles serve as guideposts to a healthy life: the Principle of Unity and the Principle of Inner Guidance.

❧ **Principle of Unity—the Greater Whole.** Like a single cell in a body, the Soul lives with the personality as a particle of energy in a great unity: the cosmos. Through the realization of our Life Plan, we automatically participate in the development of this Greater Whole. When our actions are in harmony with the purposes of the Greater Whole, it encourages us and supplies us with energy. Every action going against the interests of the larger whole interrupts this connection to the cosmic supply of energy, and will sooner or later backfire.

❧ **Principle of Inner Guidance.** The most important task in life is the development of one's Life Plan. Only by means of this can one be part of the Greater Whole and have access to the inexhaustible cosmic stream of energy. For this reason, it makes sense to pay attention to inspiration coming from one's Inner Guidance and to follow this inspiration. We should not let other people become involved in our Life Plan and should not try to influence the Life Plans of others.

Ideally, the personality should completely follow the inspiration of Inner Guidance. Then our Life Plan will be realized, bringing complete happiness, health, and contentment. Naturally, this is seldom the case.

SPIRITUAL MISUNDERSTANDINGS

Spiritual misunderstandings occur when the personality acts without consulting the inspiration of Inner Guidance. The personality perceives itself not as a part of the Greater Whole (Principle of Unity) but has the illusion of being completely independent.

Under these conditions, the personality does not turn inward (Principle of Inner Guidance), but outward. For example, it relies exclusively upon social norms or the advice of other people, thus deviating from its own Life Plan. This leads to an interruption in the cosmic energy flow and to blockages in the development of character potential. We experience these blockages as destructive behavior patterns, such as being impatient, apathetic, or domineering.

HUMAN NATURE AND THE BACH FLOWER REACTION CLUSTERS

As mentioned above, Bach defined thirty-eight negative psychic states, or distorted reaction patterns. In his thirty-eight categories, Bach defined the collective building blocks of psychic reactions in human nature. (He also identified a Flower Essence that would mediate each negative psychic state.) A crisis situation often involves the interaction of three negative states as listed in the following table.

NEGATIVE PSYCHIC STATE	MEDIATING BACH FLOWER CONCENTRATE
Feeling powerless	*Willow*
Being shocked	*Star of Bethlehem*
Doubting one's own ideas	*Cerato*

In confronting various situations, people would ideally consult their Inner Guidance to transform these fundamental building blocks into continually new sequences of reactions. But our reactions to life situations often take place unconsciously and automatically, repeating the same progression of reaction patterns over and over again. In such cases, a vicious mental cycle can develop. In the example above, the three negative psychic states often interact with one another as follows:

When I feel attacked in a given situation, I immediately feel shaken up,	*Star of Bethlehem*
and I feel like a victim,	*Willow*
because I am not entirely sure of my own stated opinion.	*Cerato*
This makes me feel more and more vulnerable.	*Star of Bethlehem, Willow*

In this book I describe these combinations of negative states as reaction clusters, along with their associated Bach Flower Concentrates (see page 122). In crisis situations, a great number of people repeatedly express identical reaction clusters in the form of negative beliefs. Taking the Bach Flower Concentrates listed for each reaction cluster mediates a reconnection with your Inner Guidance, opening the way for progress and change.

In the course of intensive work with Bach Flower Remedies and the spiritual principles of Bach Flower Therapy, a liberating feeling will gradually arise, allowing inner resistance to melt away bit by bit. Then—very often during a good conversation—an "aha! moment" will take place, and through it, a new direction can be taken toward solving the crisis at hand.

Connecting with Your Inner Guidance

Countless different methods, books, and seminars deal with this topic. In one thing they are all united: the process begins with centering.

One may speak of centering, meditating, grounding oneself, or contemplation—whatever term is used, this ultimately means turning your entire attention consciously inward and perceiving that you are entirely internally focused on yourself.

A state of deep concentration ensues, in which you lose "normal perception of time" and gain a sense of timelessness. Now the channels to your Inner Guidance are opened, and the impulses of this guidance can be received as inspiration.

But centering is not achieved solely by conscious meditation. One can also achieve it physically, through breathing, yoga, dance, or t'ai chi. Others center themselves by becoming immersed in creative activities, such as sculpting, painting, or singing. And some people find their center by cleaning their gardening tools or writing down a list of things that they want to accomplish the next day.

The unmistakable indicator of centering is that these activities, under these conditions, do not cause "mental strain" but take place effortlessly and joyfully. When one is centered, one has a feeling of being in the middle of things and of being entirely present. You should feel calm, strong in a gentle way, and should know that you have the courage necessary to handle every moment of life.

Edward Bach recommended a simple form of centering, which every person in every life situation can perform:

Every day, at the same time, sit still in a quiet place for fifteen minutes and think over the experiences of the day and of your life.

HOW CRISES UNFOLD AND
WHICH BACH FLOWERS CAN HELP

The resolution of most crises follows a familiar progression. A problem arises that simply cannot be ignored. Though we might try to deny the problem at first, it becomes so acute that denial is impossible. We don't have a clear idea of how to solve the problem, but we are afraid to lose what we *do* have by making any major change to the status quo. Gradually, though, we gain insight into the situation and stop resisting change. Finally we act upon our new insights to turn the situation around. Depending on the multifaceted nature of the crisis in question, these phases may overlap in individual cases. This can result in the temporary feeling that one is living a life of crisis.

The Anatomy of a Crisis

- **Denial phase:** I don't want to acknowledge the problem; I'm not affected by it (yet).
- **Resistance phase:** I recognize that I have a problem, but I'm afraid to change or give up my current situation.
- **Insight and perception phase:** As a result of one or several revealing experiences, I can stop resisting the need to change my situation.
- **New direction and turnaround phase:** I put my new insights and perceptions into practice.

How can I tell that I am going through a crisis?

When facing a problem, the strategies I have used successfully in the past are no longer effective. The situation escalates, and I suffer. I want to change something, but I don't know how. This makes me uncertain and fearful and undermines my self-reliance.

Feelings That Indicate a Crisis . . . and the Bach Flowers That Can Help

☐ A certain situation makes me more and more
  uncomfortable.   *Wild Oat, Beech*

☐ I feel more and more tired; I feel like I don't have
  enough energy to face the day.   *Hornbeam*

☐ I have a vague feeling of anxiety that I can't quite pin down. *Aspen*

☐ I feel as though I'm getting a raw deal.   *Heather*

☐ My thoughts keep running in circles and keep me
  awake at night.   *White Chestnut*

☐ My mind keeps wandering.   *Clematis*

☐ I feel more sensitive and unstable
  than usual.   *Holly, Gentian, Scleranthus*

☐ I am more irritable than usual.   *Impatiens*

☐ I have more trouble than usual concentrating
  on everyday tasks.   *Clematis*

What are crises good for?

In a crisis situation, remember that a crisis is a kind of rebirth. A part of your personality that was previously denied, unknown, or atrophied can now develop fully. You will become more of who you truly are. Tested by the crisis, you will become truer and stronger. Though it may be difficult to do so when you are in the middle of a real-life crisis, try to keep the following points in mind.

  ଛ This crisis is leading me out of a dead-end situation.
  ଛ This crisis will make long-needed change possible. It also
    will produce the energy I need for taking this new step. It

has been scientifically proven that a crisis situation enables us to accept new things more quickly than usual and makes it easier for us to break free from old, established behavior patterns.

❧ Once I have overcome this crisis, my psychic energy, which was blocked by this problem, will be free—as will the energy that has been blocked in all similar, earlier unresolved crises. Therefore, I will have more energy overall at my disposal.

❧ My crisis management competence is growing. This means I will be better able to deal with future crises.

Normal Reaction Patterns for the Beginning of an Acute Crisis and the Bach Flowers That Can Help

☐ I completely lose my head and fall into a panic. *Rock Rose*

☐ I try to control my fear. *Cherry Plum*

☐ I space out or mentally "check out." *Star of Bethlehem, Clematis*

☐ I feel as if I can't be objective about myself anymore. *Cherry Plum, Agrimony*

☐ I tell myself that I have to be stronger. *Rock Water*

☐ I feel that I have to change something quickly, otherwise I won't be able to tolerate it anymore. *Impatiens*

☐ I am desperately looking for a way out. *Wild Oat, Impatiens*

☐ I feel powerless, a victim of circumstances. *Willow*

☐ I get angry, either at myself or at others. *Holly*

☐ I feel that all my possibilities are exhausted, as if I'm trapped in a corner. *Sweet Chestnut*

☐ My reactions are more unstable than usual. *Scleranthus*

☐ I react more sensitively than usual.   *Impatiens*

☐ I have trouble concentrating on everyday activities.   *Clematis*

Reaction Patterns Common During the Resistance Phase and the Bach Flowers That Can Help

In this phase, almost all Bach Flower conditions can theoretically occur. The following patterns and clusters are especially common; they can change quickly and sometimes coincide.

☐ I distract myself and don't want to notice things.   *Agrimony*

☐ I don't trust myself anymore; I no longer know what I should think.   *Cerato*

☐ I am indecisive; is this really the right thing for me?   *Wild Oat*

☐ I feel helpless and abandoned.   *Heather, Willow*

☐ I criticize others or myself.   *Beech*

☐ I am incapable. I can't do anything right.   *Larch*

☐ I am angry—at myself or at others.   *Holly*

☐ I'll show them—they can't do that to me!   *Vine*

☐ I'll stick it out!   *Oak*

☐ How am I supposed to deal with this?   *Elm*

☐ Can I really do this? I just can't do this to someone!   *Pine*

☐ But it's been so nice all this time . . .   *Honeysuckle*

☐ I'm being pulled this way and that. Should I really give up the old? Is the new really any good?   *Scleranthus, Honeysuckle*

Psychic Conditions Often
Neglected in the New Orientation Phase
and the Bach Flowers That Can Help

☐ The decision has been made, but now
   I feel awful and very sad.   *Mustard*

☐ I feel exhausted.   *Olive*

☐ I still feel very vulnerable.   *Holly, Star of Bethlehem*

☐ I feel guilty toward others, believing
   they are suffering in the new situation.   *Pine*

☐ Well-meaning advice from others continues to make
   me question my decision.   *Walnut*

When you lose your strength in a crisis . . .

When you are overcome by a crisis, a great deal of psychic energy is used. It is important to act on this, so that the energy can be replenished. Do something for yourself with a very specific purpose. Reach for things that have given you strength and balance in similar past situations (for example, gardening, taking a bath, dancing, listening to music, calling an old friend, or going for a walk). The new Bach Flower Reharmony Program may also be helpful.

Where in the process should
Rescue Remedy be taken?

At the beginning of an acute crisis, Rescue Remedy—taken in a glass of water—is the best crisis treatment. Rescue Remedy is the best-known Bach Flower Remedy. A combination of Star of Bethlehem, Rock Rose, Impatiens, Cherry Plum, and Clematis, its emotionally stabilizing and psychophysically relaxing effects begin within minutes. This creates the best possible conditions for dealing with the situation and with one's personal crisis patterns.

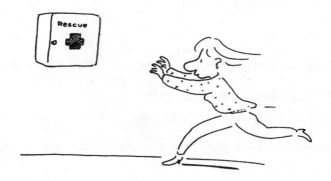

But Rescue Remedy is no substitute for Flower Therapy; at best it is a first step in this direction. When you have been overwhelmed by long-term crisis situations, as described in this book, Rescue Remedy can be taken continually, along with your individual Flower Remedies, whenever the situation escalates. (See more about Rescue Remedy on page 238.)

How to
Use This Book

In this book, you will find fifty common crisis situations and the reactions of the affected person, stated in terms of reaction clusters according to the principles of Bach Flower Therapy. Studying the reactions that other people have to common crisis situations can help you to identify your own negative belief patterns and the Bach Flower Concentrates that would be most helpful for you.

Although this sounds all well and good in theory, in practice it is usually not so easy. Accompanying therapeutic treatments may be necessary. Often enough, the right possibilities will occur to you when you are internally ready for them.

But you should not expect this book to be a patent remedy for all your current crisis situations. Rather, use it to help you recognize your own (probably deeply rooted) destructive reaction patterns more clearly and to guide you to constructive help during crises.

❦

Step 1: Read the chapter in part 1 about the crisis area that corresponds to your crisis—"Family and Children," "Partnerships and Relationships," "Career and Professional Life," "Aging," or "Other Crises"—choosing the case that comes closest to your own personal situation. Even if the case you choose is not exactly the same as your own, you probably will find behavior patterns in the given section that can be applied to your crisis. If you can't find an appropriate match, please read the other cases in the corresponding chapter.

At the beginning of a crisis, you can determine your appropriate Flower mixture to a great degree from the described cases. (When reading this book, you may notice that certain Bach Flowers are mentioned repeatedly, for example, Willow. This is part of the nature of a crisis situation. But combinations with other Flowers still yield different results.)

For the subsequent second and third mixtures, the reaction cluster section of this book will indicate the correct treatment.

Step 2: Write down all the Bach Flowers you have found. If there are a large number of Flowers, consider which Flower reactions are strongest and remove the less intense ones from the list. For this, see also page 122.

Step 3: Use the information on the Flowers chosen, especially regarding spiritual misunderstandings. (See the final chapter of the book—"The 38 Individual Bach Flower Remedies, Plus Rescue Remedy"—for information on the spiritual misunderstandings mediated by each Flower.) Consider what you can recognize and change in your current situation.

Step 4: Combine the Flowers you have chosen, which you will take for two to three weeks (see the chapter "How to Prepare Bach Flower Combinations").

Step 5: Combine this mixture with an initial empowering statement, which will accompany and lead you as a theme through the desired phase of change. Depending on your needs, this statement can always be modified.

Step 6: Evaluate what the Flower combination has done for you so far after three to four weeks, or when your remedy bottle is empty. What new steps have you taken, and what steps will you still take? How does the situation seem to you now?

Step 7: Make a new Flower mixture for this revised situation, and repeat the steps given above.

AN EXAMPLE OF A PATTERN

Step 1: In your current crisis situation, you feel exploited. The case that comes closest to this crisis situation is story number 29: "My friend sees me as nothing but a psychic dumping ground."

In this case, you identify the following reaction patterns as similar to your own:

☐ I can't hold my own against my friend's
torrent of words. *Centaury*

☐ I often feel hurt, but so far I have always put
a good face on things. *Holly, Agrimony*

☐ I am afraid to criticize my friend, for fear of
losing our friendship. *Mimulus, Chicory*

Step 2: You note the Flowers: *Centaury, Holly, Agrimony, Mimulus,* and *Chicory.*

Step 3: You study the concepts for the individual Flowers in the final chapter of the book—"The 38 Individual Bach Flower Remedies, Plus Rescue Remedy."* After dealing with psychic misunderstandings, recognize and identify them as a first step.

---

*For further information about each Bach Flower, see Mechthild Scheffer, *The Encyclopedia of Bach Flower Therapy* (Rochester, VT: Healing Arts Press, 2001) and *Mastering Bach Flower Therapies: A Guide to Diagnosis & Treatment* (Rochester, VT: Healing Arts Press, 1996).

☐ I will make myself tell my friend honestly
   that her behavior hurts me.   *Centaury, Mimulus, Agrimony, Holly*

☐ If she deserts me after this (which I can't possibly
   imagine), then it never was really a true friendship.   *Chicory*

Step 4: In this case, you combine all the Flowers to prepare a Flower combination for yourself.

Step 5: Your first empowering statement is:

☐ I can do this.   *Mimulus*

☐ I am honest.   *Agrimony*

☐ I am loved.   *Chicory*

This empowering statement changes after twelve days into:

☐ I am standing strong.   *Centaury*

☐ I feel calm.   *Agrimony*

☐ I am getting strength from the source.   *Chicory*

Step 6: After three weeks, you evaluate the situation and realize the following:

The conversation with my friend has brought us closer together. I now point it out to her when she interrupts me. For this reason, we argue more than we used to. But for this situation, I do not need a flower combination.

Step 7: Not applicable in this case.

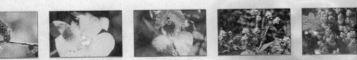

PART 1

Crisis Situations and Bach Flower Reactions: 50 Sample Cases

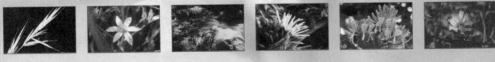

Family and Children

1. My baby wants to be breast-fed all night long. I can't stand it anymore!

"My baby wakes up every hour or two during the night and wants to be breast-fed. But my husband has to get up at 6:00 a.m. to go to work, and he needs his sleep. I have moved out of the bedroom and now sleep in the children's room, so that I can calm little Oliver right away when he wakes up.

"Another problem is that our sex life is on hold because of this. There's no question of sex, since besides being in the other bedroom, I'm hardly getting any sleep myself. And then I'm also expected to follow my mother-in-law's well-meaning advice: 'You have to let your baby cry so that his lungs will grow strong.' Or: 'You'll turn Oliver into a little tyrant if you always feed him right away.' I can't stand it anymore!"

Recommendations

1. Write down your answers to the following question: Which reactions and Flowers correspond to me? If too few reactions are found, read the other cases in this chapter.
2. Refer as necessary to the reaction clusters section of this book.
3. Read the additional steps in the "How to Use This Book" chapter.

How do I react, and what Bach Flower patterns are identifiable?

☐ Even as I'm falling asleep, I'm anxious
that the baby will cry again. *Mimulus*

☐ I feel completely at the mercy of the situation. *Willow*

☐ I am exhausted and doubting my abilities as a mother.
It seems so easy for other people. *Olive, Larch*

☐ I'm overwhelmed with guilt feelings about my husband,
since everything has become so complicated. *Pine*

☐ I know I need to get a handle on things, but sometimes
I just want to cry from exhaustion. *Oak, Olive*

☐ I try not to let others notice—especially my husband
and in-laws. Inside I am at my wits' end and often
cry in secret. *Agrimony, Sweet Chestnut*

☐ I don't know whether I can get through this situation
at all. When will there be time for me again? *Gentian, Heather*

Mimulus   *Willow*   *Olive*   *Larch*

Pine   *Oak*   *Agrimony*   *Sweet Chestnut*

Gentian   *Heather*

2. My daughter won't eat.

"My daughter Sarah (age 3) is underweight for her age, according to the pediatrician, and it's simply because she doesn't seem to like to eat. This has been a problem practically since her birth. I had too little breast milk and she didn't gain enough weight. When I began weaning her, Sarah rejected the bottle. So the subject of nourishment has been a problem for us from the beginning.

"Now Sarah is extremely picky about what she likes and doesn't like. I always try to please her and think about it almost constantly—what I will buy, what I'll cook that Sarah will like.

"When she does eat, it is only small portions. I'm always trying all kinds of tricks to get her to eat more. I don't even care what it is—if she would eat ice cream three times a day, at least she'd be consuming calories.

"Everyone thinks she's too thin, and I can't bear to hear it anymore! I don't know what more I can do."

Recommendations

1. Write down your answers to the following question: "Which reactions and Flowers correspond to me?" If too few reactions are found, read the other cases in this chapter.
2. Refer as necessary to the reaction clusters section of this book.
3. Read the additional steps in the "How to Use This Book" chapter.

How do I react, and what Bach Flower patterns are identifiable?

☐ I am fixated on the subject of food, and I can't
stop thinking about it.   *White Chestnut*

☐ I am under pressure because so many people
think my daughter needs to eat more.   *Cherry Plum*

☐ I am putting constant "gentle" pressure on my
daughter, and thereby causing her stress. *Chicory*

☐ I have extreme guilt feelings because I wasn't
able to breast-feed my daughter sufficiently. I think
this is still hanging over us. *Pine*

☐ I want so much to put everything right, but I think
I'm a failure as a mother. I often find myself
completely despairing about all this. *Larch, Sweet Chestnut*

☐ I see myself as stuck in a vicious circle—it's like
a power game, and I can't find my way out. *Vine, Chestnut Bud*

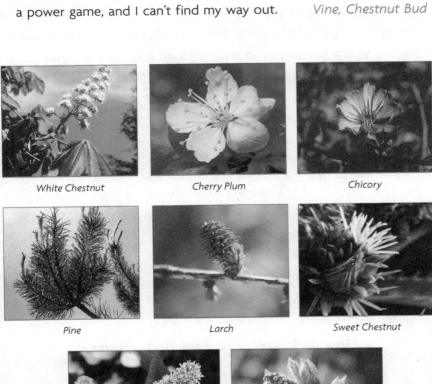

White Chestnut

Cherry Plum

Chicory

Pine

Larch

Sweet Chestnut

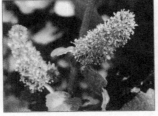

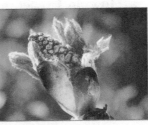

Vine

Chestnut Bud

3. My child always wants to be the center of attention. Nobody wants to invite us over anymore.

"No matter where we go, or who visits us, my four-year-old son makes a disturbance. Whether in the company of adults or other children, Kevin clowns around, acts silly, always wants to be the center of attention, does whatever he wants, and constantly provokes me. He simply won't behave. When he's reprimanded, he reacts by getting even wilder, more rambunctious, and more aggressive.

"I really wish my husband would step in and set some boundaries for our son. But he leaves me to handle the situation, and it feels as if the entire burden is on me.

"What strikes me the most is that no one invites us over anymore: the mothers' group that I had really enjoyed told me that Kevin disrupts the others with his behavior. They say I should come back when Kevin finally behaves like other children.

"Now I feel even more alone with my problems. Something has got to be done about Kevin."

Recommendations

1. Write down your answers to the following question: "Which reactions and Flowers correspond to me?" If too few reactions are found, read the other cases in this chapter.
2. Refer as necessary to the reaction clusters section of this book.
3. Read the additional steps in the "How to Use This Book" chapter.

How do I react, and what Bach Flower patterns are identifiable?

☐ Even first thing in the morning, I'm anxious about power struggles with my child.   *Mimulus*

☐ I'm so angry at my child that I yell at him constantly.   *Holly*

☐ I scold, threaten, punish—but it does no good. I can't see
any way out of this out-of-control situation.   *Vine, Sweet Chestnut*

☐ I'm so irritated that I have no tolerance left. I have
emotionally distanced myself from my child.   *Beech, Water Violet*

☐ I'm embarrassed in front of others, and feel I have
failed as a mother.   *Larch*

☐ Since no one supports me, not even my husband, I feel
abandoned and no longer equal to the responsibility.   *Heather, Elm*

☐ Sometimes I feel downright hateful toward my child.
Then I naturally have strong guilt feelings, because a
mother shouldn't feel this way.   *Holly, Pine*

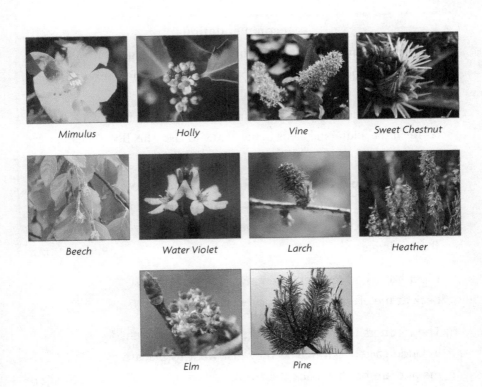

| Mimulus | Holly | Vine | Sweet Chestnut |

| Beech | Water Violet | Larch | Heather |

| Elm | Pine |

4. My daughter (age 4) is in kindergarten. The separation is difficult for both of us.

"For four weeks now Nicole has been in kindergarten, but each morning she cries a little when I drop her off. The teachers tell me she cheers up quickly, but are they telling me the truth? Nicole is still so little, and she can't explain to me what happens in kindergarten and what she doesn't like.

"On the other hand, I can't spend the whole day worrying about her because I've gone back to my part-time job as an accountant.

"I have only bad memories of my own kindergarten days; I felt abandoned and unhappy, and I cried a lot. I wonder if I'm projecting my feelings from back then onto my daughter, because Nicole actually enjoys being around other children."

Recommendations

1. Write down your answers to the following question: "Which reactions and Flowers correspond to me?" If too few reactions are found, read the other cases in this chapter.
2. Refer as necessary to the reaction clusters section of this book.
3. Read the additional steps in the "How to Use This Book" chapter.

How do I react, and what Bach Flower patterns are identifiable?

☐ It is very difficult for me to leave my child at
the kindergarten. *Red Chestnut*

☐ I feel like a bad mother when my child looks sadly
back at me after I kiss her good-bye. *Pine*

☐ The teachers tell me things are going well for my child
in kindergarten, but maybe they just want to placate
me and are holding back the truth. *Gentian*

☐ I can't fully enjoy the things I do while my child is at kindergarten, because I have a guilty conscience.

Pine

☐ I often think back on my own unhappy kindergarten days.

Honeysuckle

☐ I'm concerned that I may be worrying too much about my daughter and projecting my own memories onto her.

Cerato, Red Chestnut

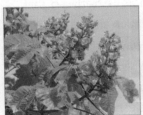

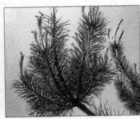
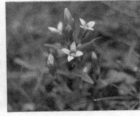

Red Chestnut   *Pine*   *Gentian*

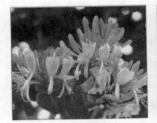
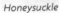
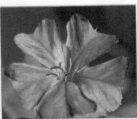

Honeysuckle   *Cerato*

5. Since my divorce, I have made sure my child (age 6) has everything he could possibly need. Am I neglecting myself?

"Since the divorce, my only concern has been my son, Jonathan. My ex-husband is in a new relationship and no longer has any contact with us. Right now I am there only for my son, and my own needs and interests have fallen by the wayside. I am completely obsessed with the idea of being both father and mother to him at the same time.

"I hardly ever go out any more, and a new relationship is unthinkable for me. I mostly only meet with other people secretly, so that my son won't feel left out. I pamper my son too much and let him get away with a great deal. Jonathan always gets his way.

"Now he even wants to fall asleep in bed with me every night, although I prefer sleeping alone. I badly need an undisturbed night's rest. I agonize over whether I can dare to be so selfish as to insist that he stay in his own room at night."

Recommendations

1. Write down your answers to the following question: "Which reactions and Flowers correspond to me?" If too few reactions are found, read the other cases in this chapter.
2. Refer as necessary to the reaction clusters section of this book.
3. Read the additional steps in the "How to Use This Book" chapter.

How do I react, and what Bach Flower patterns are identifiable?

☐ The desire for my son not to be hurt by the
divorce dominates everything.   *Rock Water, Agrimony*

☐ I feel guilty, as if I have taken my son's father away
from him, and I feel selfish whenever I think of myself at all.   *Pine*

☐ I often feel isolated and alone.   *Water Violet*

☐ I can't say no when my son asks me for something. *Centaury*

☐ The situation overwhelms me. I feel helpless and
powerless. *Willow, Elm*

☐ I feel restricted and trapped in a situation I can't
change. *Sweet Chestnut*

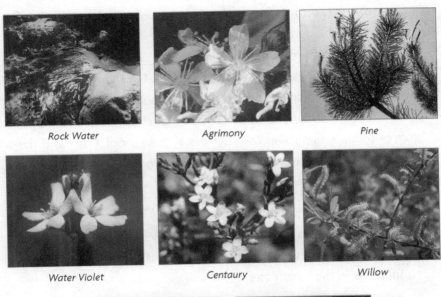

Rock Water   *Agrimony*   *Pine*

Water Violet   *Centaury*   *Willow*

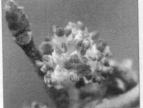
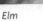
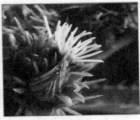

Elm   *Sweet Chestnut*

6. Switching schools: yes or no?

"My son is seven years old and in the first grade. He is a very intelligent child, able to read since he was three years old and also especially skillful at math. Despite this, the teacher tells me he's not ready for school.

"The problem is that he is restless and dreamy, always does whatever he wants, and so is usually not very organized. When he does his homework, it takes him forever to complete what is required. But if I'm strict with him, things go even worse.

"It seems to me that the teacher doesn't understand his special abilities, and I am in favor of switching schools. But the whole family is against it. They all think he needs to see it through and learn to fit in.

"Now I have to decide whether to find a school better suited for him or to leave him to his own devices at this school. I feel as if the remainder of his school years are dependent on my decision."

Recommendations

1. Write down your answers to the following question: "Which reactions and Flowers correspond to me?" If too few reactions are found, read the other cases in this chapter.
2. Refer as necessary to the reaction clusters section of this book.
3. Read the additional steps in the "How to Use This Book" chapter.

How do I react, and what Bach Flower patterns are identifiable?

☐ I keep trying to be stricter, insisting that my son do his homework in an organized manner, but this only leads to quarrels and tears.   *Vine*

☐ When he cries, I reproach myself for being so mean.   *Pine*

☐ Then I once again become very sympathetic and
feel myself torn between discipline and empathy. *Scleranthus*

☐ I doubt my own abilities as a mother, and I allow
my family to make me uncertain about whether
I am truly in favor of switching schools. *Larch, Walnut*

☐ I am angry at the teacher and also angry at my
husband, who never takes my side. *Holly*

☐ I'm afraid that my child is not getting the right
kind of start to his future education. *Mimulus, Gentian*

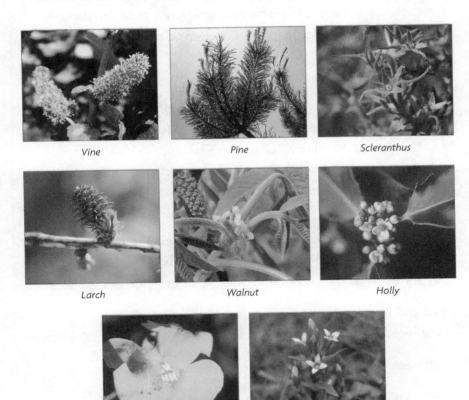

Vine   *Pine*   *Scleranthus*

Larch   *Walnut*   *Holly*

Mimulus   *Gentian*

7. As a single mother, I'm totally overextended.

"Klaus and I got divorced. He remarried and I didn't. Our daughter—now ten years old—stayed with me. The multiple stresses of child, household, and my job as a travel agent are draining me. Each morning when I get up, I am already fearful that I won't be able to handle all the work. It always (just barely) gets done, but I am totally exhausted and worn out at the end of the day and not a happy mother for my child.

"On weekends I have to clean the house and desperately need to take a bit of a rest. I don't have much motivation to do anything with my daughter. Of course this makes her sad and gives me a guilty conscience. Perhaps I should have looked around for a new daddy for her, but it's too late for that now. I've given up on it."

Recommendations

1. Write down your answers to the following question: "Which reactions and Flowers correspond to me?" If too few reactions are found, read the other cases in this chapter.
2. Refer as necessary to the reaction clusters section of this book.
3. Read the additional steps in the "How to Use This Book" chapter.

How do I react, and what Bach Flower patterns are identifiable?

☐ I feel totally at the end of my rope; it's all too much. *Olive*

☐ When I wake up in the morning, the day ahead of me looks like a mountain I have to climb. *Hornbeam*

☐ This bothers me—after all, other people manage just fine. *Larch*

☐ All I am doing is functioning. I'm unable to take pleasure in things. I don't even feel anything anymore. *Oak*

☐ No matter how hard I try, I can't do right by my daughter or by myself. Things can't go on this way! *Sweet Chestnut*

☐ I would really like some help, but I
can't get up the nerve to ask anyone. *Mimulus, Water Violet*

☐ Somehow, I did everything wrong. I probably
don't even deserve a better life. *Beech, Willow, Wild Rose*

☐ I've given up trying to find a partner who will
really support me. *Wild Rose*

Olive

Hornbeam

Larch

Oak

Sweet Chestnut

Mimulus

Water Violet

Beech

Willow

Wild Rose

8. My son (age 14) does nothing but sit at the computer.

"As the single mother of a fourteen-year-old son, I am going through a crisis: for quite a while now, Luke does nothing but sit at the computer. I can't do anything with him—his grandparents are already rather hurt by his behavior—and he hardly does anything with his friends anymore. He's stopped going to Judo class, and he seems not to take an interest in anything. I don't know what he's doing at the computer all this time, because he shuts himself in his room and is inaccessible.

"I'm really worried about what this will lead to. I would like to bring him to a psychologist, but Luke refuses. The only thing I ever hear from him is 'Leave me alone!' Sometimes I find this very hurtful, all the more so because as a mother I have to take responsibility when things aren't going well. Sometimes I think that I should be more strict and threaten to take away his allowance."

Recommendations

1. Write down your answers to the following question: "Which reactions and Flowers correspond to me?" If too few reactions are found, read the other cases in this chapter.
2. Refer as necessary to the reaction clusters section of this book.
3. Read the additional steps in the "How to Use This Book" chapter.

How do I react, and what Bach Flower patterns are identifiable?

☐ I am very unsure as to how I should act. Every person tells me to do something different: "Wait it out," "Do something now" . . . I just don't know anymore! *Cerato, Scleranthus*

☐ I constantly think and worry about my son, so I'm very anxious. *Red Chestnut*

☐ I respond by feeling hurt and offended, because I want only what's best for him. *Holly, Chicory*

☐ Although I know that my son is hurting himself by doing this,
I can't bring myself to act firmly. *Centaury, Vine*

☐ I'm worried that my son will become an outsider and that I will feel
like a terrible mother because I didn't do anything. *Mimulus, Pine*

☐ As a single parent, the whole burden is on me,
and I feel overwhelmed by this situation. *Elm, Willow*

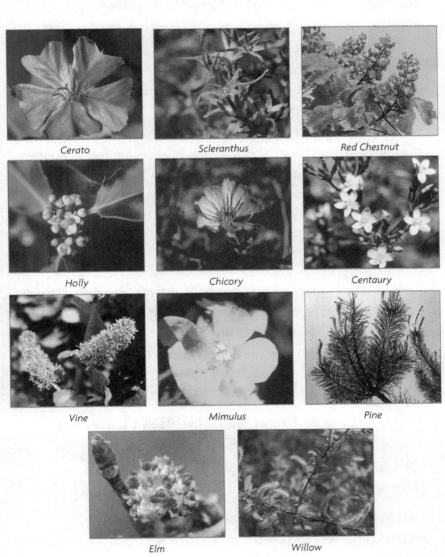

Cerato	Scleranthus	Red Chestnut
Holly	Chicory	Centaury
Vine	Mimulus	Pine
Elm	Willow	

9. Am I a good enough mother for my blended family?

"After my divorce four years ago, I found a new partner who had a son, then ten, and a daughter, then twelve (the same age as my own son), from his previous marriage. The problem, as with any blended family, is that we haven't all gone through various important developmental phases together. So now I have to absorb, at "high speed" so to speak, everything that affected the "new children" while growing up. Ultimately, it feels as though a huge responsibility has landed on my shoulders.

"At the same time, I'm worried about being seen as the wicked stepmother who cross-examines the children and asks too many questions. I am under constant pressure because I'm always picturing the harmonious family ideal.

"But the reality is completely different. For a long time I had the feeling that a real mother-daughter relationship had developed between my stepdaughter and me. But now she keeps saying she wants to go back to her real mother. This hurts me a great deal. What am I doing wrong?"

Recommendations

1. Write down your answers to the following question: "Which reactions and Flowers correspond to me?" If too few reactions are found, read the other cases in this chapter.
2. Refer as necessary to the reaction clusters section of this book.
3. Read the additional steps in the "How to Use This Book" chapter.

How do I react, and what Bach Flower patterns are identifiable?

☐ I feel disappointed and hurt by my stepdaughter's
behavior.   *Holly, Chicory*

☐ I am completely drained, because I always have to be
on guard and alert so that things won't go wrong.   *Chicory, Olive*

☐ Sometimes I feel that I'm not equal to my role as mother in a blended family. *Elm*

☐ I put pressure on myself because of my conception of an ideal family. *Rock Water*

☐ I am worried that the children will see me as the wicked stepmother. *Mimulus, Larch*

☐ My husband and I often quarrel because we have different ideas about how to raise children. These fights hurt me a great deal. *Agrimony, Holly*

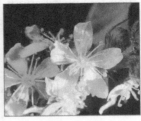

Holly

Chicory

Olive

Elm

Rock Water

Mimulus

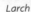

Larch

Agrimony

10. My family is taking advantage of me.

"I am forty-four. My children are my first priority, so there is no time left for me. My son is a student and lives in a shared apartment, but every weekend he brings his dirty laundry home for me to wash. My two teenage daughters invite their friends over to our house nearly every day. I am expected to cook for all of them, so I slave away in the kitchen and it doesn't occur to anyone to help me clean up.

"All day long I hear, 'Can you do this? . . . Can you do that? . . . Mom, did you do this yet? . . .' When I need help, no one is there for me. They all take it for granted that I will be totally at their disposal.

"Keeping up with this strenuous workload is exhausting. I've been trying to please everybody, but now I'm feeling overwhelmed by it all."

Recommendations

1. Write down your answers to the following question: Which reactions and Flowers correspond to me? If too few reactions are found, read the other cases in this chapter.
2. Refer as necessary to the reaction clusters section of this book.
3. Read the additional steps in the "How to Use This Book" chapter.

How do I react, and what Bach Flower patterns are identifiable?

☐ I am always irascible and nervous. I often yell at my
children, then feel guilty about it later.   *Impatiens, Holly, Pine*

☐ I often feel as though I'm being Mother Teresa for everyone. They seem to feel as if they can just pile everything up on me.   *Willow*

☐ Sometimes I function like a robot, holding myself
back with gritted teeth.   *Oak, Rock Water*

☐ I often feel attacked by others, and I wish criticism
didn't hurt me so much.   *Holly*

☐ I can't say no, because I always want to make
things right.   *Centaury, Agrimony*

☐ It is difficult for me to neglect doing something, or to
delegate it to someone else.   *Elm*

☐ When I need help, no one is there.   *Heather, Willow*

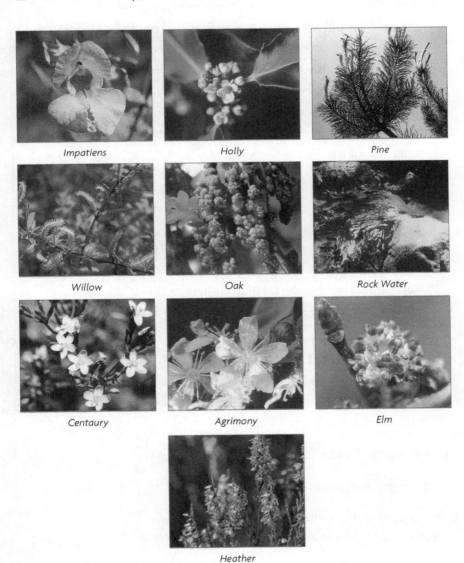

Impatiens   *Holly*   *Pine*

Willow   *Oak*   *Rock Water*

Centaury   *Agrimony*   *Elm*

Heather

11. Lena (age 14): No one understands me or my world.

"My parents' lifestyle is so bourgeois. And they expect me to be just as boring as they are: always eating dinner together at the same time, then crashing in front of the tube for the evening. I'd rather stay in my room and talk on the phone with my best friend or hang out with my friends at the youth club. At least they understand me.

"When I go out wearing a top that shows my belly button, my mom always flips out. It doesn't do any good to explain to her that everyone dresses this way. Recently I got this amazing tattoo on my lower back—at least she can't take *that* away from me.

"My parents just don't want to understand me. They don't make the least bit of effort. My mom has even threatened to speak to my teachers about me. I think that's just plain rude!"

Recommendations

1. Write down your answers to the following question: "Which reactions and Flowers correspond to me?" If too few reactions are found, read the other cases in this chapter.
2. Refer as necessary to the reaction clusters section of this book.
3. Read the additional steps in the "How to Use This Book" chapter.

How do I react, and what Bach Flower patterns are identifiable?

☐ My parents still treat me like a child, even
   though I feel entirely grown-up.   *Walnut, Willow*

☐ I feel rejected and misunderstood.   *Willow*

☐ I get angry and yell at my parents.   *Holly, Cherry Plum*

☐ If my parents think they can tell me what to do,
   they're wrong.   *Vine*

☐ If they keep this up, they'll see. They'll get
what they're asking for.

Holly, Vine

☐ Sometimes I just slam the door, because I can't
be bothered listening to my mother's nagging
anymore.

Beech, Water Violet

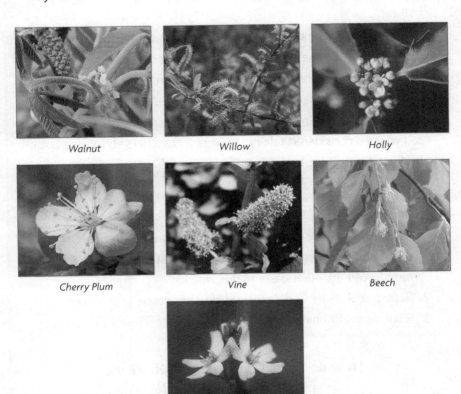

Walnut *Willow* *Holly*

Cherry Plum *Vine* *Beech*

Water Violet

12. Judith (age 37): I no longer understand my fourteen-year-old daughter's world.

"My daughter has changed so much recently that it frightens me. She used to be such a sweet child, but now she's always defiant and won't take any advice from us. Whatever I say, for her it's nothing but 'bullshit.'

"And the way she dresses! I don't want her to look so slutty. And I don't care if it's the way all the other girls are dressing. I can't get through to my daughter at all anymore. When she was younger, she always shared her secrets with me. Now she confides only in her friends, who are a terrible influence on her.

"I've even considered talking with Lena's teachers about her, but if she found out about it, she would be furious."

Recommendations

1. Write down your answers to the following question: "Which reactions and Flowers correspond to me?" If too few reactions are found, read the other cases in this chapter.
2. Refer as necessary to the reaction clusters section of this book.
3. Read the additional steps in the "How to Use This Book" chapter.

How do I react, and what Bach Flower patterns are identifiable?

☐ I completely disapprove of the way my daughter
dresses every day.   *Beech*

☐ I feel completely overwhelmed by raising my daughter,
and I don't know what to do anymore.   *Sweet Chestnut*

☐ I worry about my daughter's future.   *Red Chestnut*

☐ I am afraid of losing control over my daughter.   *Vine, Mimulus*

☐ I feel like I can't even stand up to my own underage
daughter. To keep things pleasant and harmonious,
I often just give in to her. *Agrimony, Centaury*

☐ I'm disappointed and jealous that my daughter shares what's
important to her only with her friends now. *Gentian, Chicory*

☐ All the effort I made to bring her up properly
is being lost. How can I stop this? *Chicory*

☐ I feel rejected and misunderstood. *Willow*

Beech

Sweet Chestnut

Red Chestnut

Vine

Mimulus

Agrimony

Centaury

Gentian

Chicory

Willow

13. My son (age 19) doesn't want to live at home anymore.

"My son has started university and has now suddenly confronted me with his decision to move in with a school friend—in the same city where we live. He says he wants to be independent from me. Since I am a single parent, and was always very devoted to him, this is like getting the rug pulled out from under me.

"We always did a lot of things together, went bicycling on the weekends, went to movies, went out to eat, and obviously also went on vacations together. Alex was the center of my life.

"When people criticized me for making him into too much of a mama's boy, I always blew it off. Besides him, I have hardly any friends. Am I now supposed to visit him every weekend with a bag full of groceries and wash his clothes for him? Or would this be a mistake?"

Recommendations

1. Write down your answers to the following question: "Which reactions and Flowers correspond to me?" If too few reactions are found, read the other cases in this chapter.
2. Refer as necessary to the reaction clusters section of this book.
3. Read the additional steps in the "How to Use This Book" chapter.

How do I react, and what Bach Flower patterns are identifiable?

☐ The shock has paralyzed me; I'm unable to do anything.   *Star of Bethlehem*

☐ As a mother, it's difficult for me to stay out of my son's life. I don't want to lose my influence.   *Chicory*

☐ I absolutely have to stop being dependent on my son.   *Red Chestnut*

☐ I feel so horribly abandoned. Now I have no one left
to talk to.   *Heather*

☐ Sometimes I think about all the things I've done for
my son—and now he's so ungrateful!   *Chicory*

☐ I have a feeling of emptiness, and I wonder what
on earth I'm going to do with myself.   *Wild Oat, Cerato*

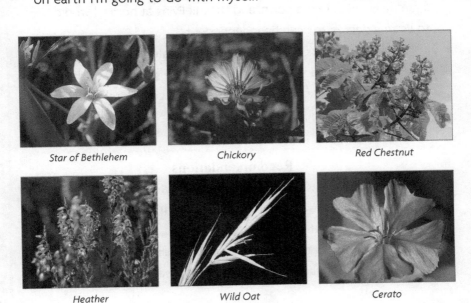

Star of Bethlehem   *Chickory*   *Red Chestnut*

Heather   *Wild Oat*   *Cerato*

14. I have become unexpectedly pregnant in the middle of college. What should I do?

"Tom and I met in college. I was in my third semester studying German and education. He was in his fifth semester studying law. Now I've found out I'm seven-weeks pregnant.

"Tom is living on student loans, and there's no way he can support a family. He lives in the dorm, and I'm still living at home. I would like to get my degree so I can be independent.

"Everything points against having a baby at this time. Tom is no help in making the decision as to whether we should keep the baby; he says I've got to know that for myself. I feel completely thrown off track, and I have no idea what to do."

Recommendations

1. Write down your answers to the following question: "Which reactions and Flowers correspond to me?" If too few reactions are found, read the other cases in this chapter.
2. Refer as necessary to the reaction clusters section of this book.
3. Read the additional steps in the "How to Use This Book" chapter.

How do I react, and what Bach Flower patterns are identifiable?

☐ I feel totally overwhelmed by the situation and can't decide whether to keep the baby, because the arguments for and against it keep going around in my head.   *Elm, Scleranthus*

☐ Actually I would be glad to have a baby, but I'm scared about the idea of quitting school.   *Mimulus*

☐ I'm very disappointed with my boyfriend, who is
leaving me totally alone in making the decision about
whether to become a mother.   *Gentian*

☐ Will I be able to take responsibility for a child?
Or is it better to concentrate on my studies and
my own needs? If I decide not to keep the baby,
will I be plagued by guilt?   *Walnut, Pine*

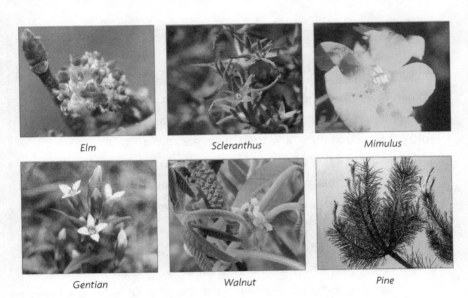

Elm   *Scleranthus*   *Mimulus*

Gentian   *Walnut*   *Pine*

Partnerships and Relationships

15. I always fall in love with the wrong man.

"When I met Xavier, he claimed he was about to be divorced from his wife. I should have paid better attention, because another man had told me the same thing, and then never got divorced.

"Once again, I had fallen in love with the wrong man. This always happens to me, because each time it's a man who is not actually available. And each time, a long period of suffering is guaranteed.

"But now I simply don't want it anymore. I ask myself: 'Why does this keep happening to me? Why am I always attracted to men with whom I can't have a normal relationship?'

"I wonder whether Xavier will make the final decision after another year. I'd like to say, 'Choose either your wife or me!' But I'm also afraid of losing him and wonder if it's better to have a sad ending than to have sadness without end."

Recommendations

1. Write down your answers to the following question: "Which reactions and Flowers correspond to me?" If too few reactions are found, read the other cases in this chapter.
2. Refer as necessary to the reaction clusters section of this book.
3. Read the additional steps in the "How to Use This Book" chapter.

How do I react, and what Bach Flower patterns are identifiable?

☐ I feel that fate has treated me unjustly. I feel very alone
because I don't have a man by my side in day-to-day life.   *Willow*

☐ I wonder whether I'm worth it, for a man to go
to the trouble of leaving his wife for me.   *Larch, Pine*

☐ I secretly doubt whether I would truly be happy having a steady
partner at my side day after day.   *Cerato, Water Violet*

☐ On the other hand, I'm jealous and feel abandoned when
he tells me he's going on vacation with his family.   *Holly, Willow*

☐ I wonder: Do I outwardly appear more undemanding and strong
than I actually am, so that men believe I just want to have some fun
for a little while, as they do?   *Beech, Water Violet*

☐ Sometimes I think I'm afraid to get deeply involved with
someone. What would happen if I got hurt or
he left me?   *Mimulus, Cerato, Agrimony*

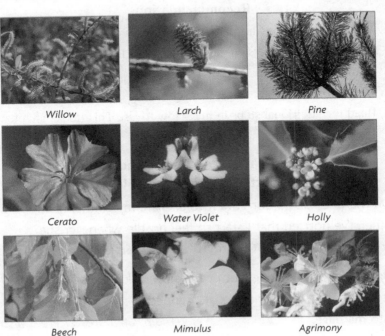

Willow   Larch   Pine

Cerato   Water Violet   Holly

Beech   Mimulus   Agrimony

16. It's difficult for me to commit myself to a relationship.

"We were invited to spend Christmas with Sabrina's parents. I was scared that she would take this opportunity to introduce me as her new partner. All my alarms were sounding! My old conflict between the desire for emotional closeness and the fear of losing my freedom came back in full force.

"I'm forty-five years old and still a bachelor, but I'm beginning to feel more and more like an outsider, and starting to doubt whether my freedom is worth the price. So far, every time a relationship has gotten too close, I've either backed out or alienated my girlfriend so as to get rid of her. Once I'm alone again, I feel lonely and rejected. This continues until I get into a new relationship.

"Is this going to go on forever? Or should I take the risk and spend Christmas with my new girlfriend and her family, giving the signal that it's a committed relationship?"

Recommendations

1. Write down your answers to the following question: "Which reactions and Flowers correspond to me?" If too few reactions are found, read the other cases in this chapter.
2. Refer as necessary to the reaction clusters section of this book.
3. Read the additional steps in the "How to Use This Book" chapter.

How do I react, and what Bach Flower patterns are identifiable?

☐ On the one hand, I don't want to alienate my girlfriend, but on the other, I've noticed that I start to feel hostile whenever she brings up the topic of Christmas. *Scleranthus, Cherry Plum*

☐ I know I'm overreacting, but I can't stop making this association of "Christmas equals trapped into marriage." *Vervain, Clematis, White Chestnut*

☐ Secretly, I feel that my girlfriend coerces me, and
I'm afraid of being dominated by her.   *Willow, Holly*

☐ If I commit to my girlfriend now, I'm afraid of
losing the opportunity to meet someone else
who is even more compatible with me.   *Wild Oat, Mimulus*

☐ Once I've ended a relationship, I feel like an outsider
who doesn't really belong anywhere and about whom
no one cares.   *Heather, Willow, Water Violet*

☐ I'm reluctant to talk with my girlfriend about my inner conflict,
because I'm worried I will scare and disappoint her if
I'm honest about it.   *Agrimony, Holly, Mimulus*

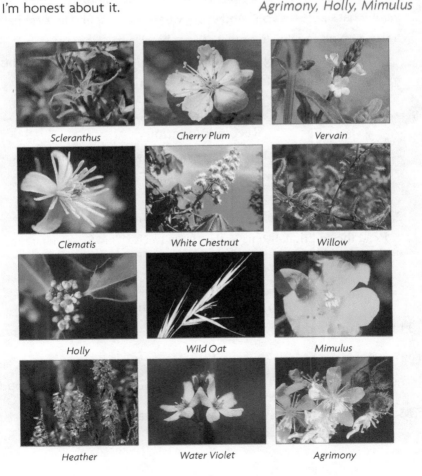

Scleranthus	*Cherry Plum*	*Vervain*
Clematis	*White Chestnut*	*Willow*
Holly	*Wild Oat*	*Mimulus*
Heather	*Water Violet*	*Agrimony*

17. Does my husband belong to his extended family, or to me?

"When I met Ralph, I knew how close he was to his family. Even on our first date, he talked constantly about his parents and siblings. I thought it was great at the time, because as an only child I had always wanted a bigger family. But after our son, James, was born, I realized that being part of such a big clan also has disadvantages.

"My mother-in-law is constantly coming over and giving me unsolicited advice. Also my two sisters-in-law, both of whom have their own children, are always showing off what perfect wives and mothers they are—even in front of Ralph. When I complain to Ralph about this, he defends them, saying, 'Don't worry about them, they only want what's best for you!' And every weekend we spend at least half a day with his family. He simply cannot break away from his clan.

"Christmas is coming, and Ralph can't get up the courage to tell his mother we'd rather celebrate the holidays on our own."

Recommendations

1. Write down your answers to the following question: "Which reactions and Flowers correspond to me?" If too few reactions are found, read the other cases in this chapter.
2. Refer as necessary to the reaction clusters section of this book.
3. Read the additional steps in the "How to Use This Book" chapter.

How do I react, and what Bach Flower patterns are identifiable?

☐ I feel patronized by my husband's family.   *Willow, Larch*

☐ I'm disappointed that my husband doesn't understand
how I feel.   *Gentian*

☐ Sometimes I think my husband is very immature.   *Beech*

☐ I feel incompetent and sometimes see myself as the
black sheep of the family.   *Larch, Willow*

☐ I feel like I can't assert my own ideas against this
huge family's overwhelming power.   *Centaury, Walnut*

☐ I am more upset about my in-laws
than I reveal.   *Holly, Agrimony, Cherry Plum*

Willow

Larch

Gentian

Beech

Centaury

Walnut

Holly

Agrimony

18. My husband wants more sex than I do.

"Why can't we just cuddle and hold each other sometimes? No, that's impossible for us. Whenever we touch, it inevitably leads to sex. Carl thinks this is completely normal.

"It's not that I'm not attracted to him, but sometimes I'd like to be able to enjoy some affection just by itself, without sex. It would also reassure me that good sex isn't the only reason Carl loves me—that he also enjoys just being close and feeling our connectedness.

"When I reject his sexual advances, I am afraid of losing him."

Recommendations

1. Write down your answers to the following question: "Which reactions and Flowers correspond to me?" If too few reactions are found, read the other cases in this chapter.
2. Refer as necessary to the reaction clusters section of this book.
3. Read the additional steps in the "How to Use This Book" chapter.

How do I react, and what Bach Flower patterns are identifiable?

☐ I have always had trouble saying "no" to things.   *Centaury*

☐ I'm afraid my husband will cheat on me if he
   doesn't get regular sex from me.   *Mimulus, Chicory*

☐ I feel guilty because I am not as passionate
   as he would like.   *Pine*

☐ I'm scared that my husband will become frustrated
   with me and that our day-to-day relationship
   will suffer.   *Chicory, Mimulus*

☐ Should I follow the example of my mother, who
believes sex is something you just have to
suffer through in silence? *Honeysuckle, Chicory*

☐ I don't know how to make it clear to my husband
that I have different needs from his. *Cerato, Walnut*

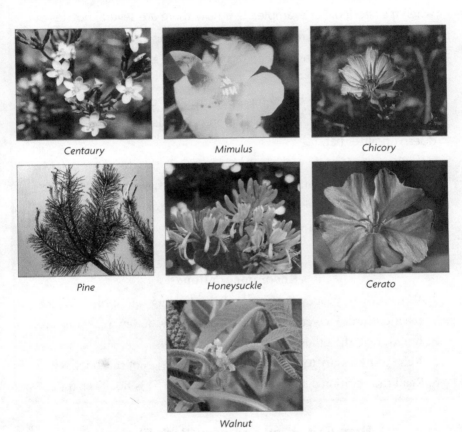

Centaury

Mimulus

Chicory

Pine

Honeysuckle

Cerato

Walnut

19. I have too low a priority in our relationship.

"My husband always does whatever he wants. He always has time for other people. He goes out for beers with his coworkers and helps the neighbors take down trees, but if I ask him to mow the lawn, he says, 'I'll get to it,' but never does. He only helps when he wants to, not when it's needed. For example, right now there are several bottles of mineral water on the floor that he's been meaning to take down to the cellar for days. When I keep reminding him about it, I seem like a nag, even to myself.

"To avoid seeming bad-tempered, I usually choose to say nothing. Actually I feel like I am walking on eggshells all the time, but he doesn't realize that.

"When I try to talk with my husband about this, he shuts off. My patience is slowly wearing down. I never would have imagined a functioning partnership this way. What I really want to do is present him with the decision: 'Either you change or I leave you!'"

Recommendations

1. Write down your answers to the following question: "Which reactions and Flowers correspond to me?" If too few reactions are found, read the other cases in this chapter.
2. Refer as necessary to the reaction clusters section of this book.
3. Read the additional steps in the "How to Use This Book" chapter.

How do I react, and what Bach Flower patterns are identifiable?

☐ I inwardly reproach my husband because I do a great deal for our relationship but he gives nothing back.   *Chicory*

☐ Sometimes I think we're simply not compatible because we have too many differences.   *Gentian*

☐ I'm sad that my husband doesn't respect my
wishes, and I feel exploited. *Willow, Gentian*

☐ I try to tell him what I mean, but he doesn't
understand me. Then I doubt myself and wonder
if I'm overreacting. *Cerato, Larch*

☐ Just to keep things peaceful, I always try to
hide my disappointment. *Agrimony*

☐ I often fume internally, fantasizing about what a
mess he would be in if I left him. *Cherry Plum, Holly*

☐ It hurts me that my husband cannot talk with
me openly about our problems. *Heather*

Chicory

Gentian

Willow

Cerato

Larch

Agrimony

Cherry Plum

Holly

Heather

20. Should I confess my infidelity?

"My husband, Max, bought me a ski vacation as a present, and I used his generosity shamelessly when I went to a resort with one of my girlfriends.

"Normally I have things well under control, but this one incident quickly turned into a soap opera. In one of the ski lodges we met a bronzed ski instructor whom I found extremely attractive. Perhaps alcohol was a factor, but in any event we ended up in my room a few hours later.

"For me it was just a one-night stand. Even the next morning, when my girlfriend gave me a knowing glance, I was already ashamed. Max doesn't know anything about it, but I'm constantly wavering between confessing it and keeping silent forever. I am haunted by uncertainty as to whether he suspects something or whether my girlfriend has snitched on me. My bad conscience plagues me so much that I would rather just tell him about my indiscretion, but I am too cowardly. You never know how a man will react to such a confession!"

Recommendations

1. Write down your answers to the following question: "Which reactions and Flowers correspond to me?" If too few reactions are found, read the other cases in this chapter.
2. Refer as necessary to the reaction clusters section of this book.
3. Read the additional steps in the "How to Use This Book" chapter.

How do I react, and what Bach Flower patterns are identifiable?

☐ I'm surprised at myself that
I cheated so readily. *Beech, Star of Bethlehem*

☐ I can never allow myself to make such a mistake again and must
behave better in the future. *Rock Water, Cherry Plum*

☐ I'm afraid to tell my husband about my
infidelity, because I don't know how he will react. *Mimulus*

☐ I am afraid that my husband suspects something
already or that he might be told something. *Aspen, Holly*

☐ I feel that I have abused my husband's trust in me. *Pine*

☐ Although this happened a long time ago, my
thoughts keep running in circles about whether
to tell him. *White Chestnut*

Beech

Star of Bethlehem

Rock Water

Cherry Plum

Mimulus

Aspen

Holly

Pine

White Chestnut

21. I can't stand being in a long-distance relationship anymore.

"Roland and I met last year on vacation. He works for a big company, and I manage a hotel in another city. Because of this we see each other only on weekends—sometimes at his place, sometimes at mine. Normally we talk on the phone each evening.

"But when I can't reach him, I immediately become mistrustful because Roland's ex-wife also lives in his city. Then I go through a whole series of imagined fears in my mind, thinking he's not really into it and will end our relationship sooner or later.

"When we see each other on weekends, he has to keep reassuring me about how much he loves me and pay constant attention to me. But at the same time, I can see that I'm getting on his nerves and that he is distancing himself emotionally."

Recommendations

1. Write down your answers to the following question: "Which reactions and Flowers correspond to me?" If too few reactions are found, read the other cases in this chapter.
2. Refer as necessary to the reaction clusters section of this book.
3. Read the additional steps in the "How to Use This Book" chapter.

How do I react, and what Bach Flower patterns are identifiable?

☐ I can't stop worrying that my boyfriend will
cheat on me and leave me.   *White Chestnut, Willow*

☐ Even small things make me mistrustful and jealous, for example,
when I can't reach him immediately on the phone.   *Holly*

☐ Sometimes I wait for hours for him to call,
and I can't concentrate on anything else.   *Red Chestnut*

☐ On weekends I expect my boyfriend to
devote himself to me exclusively.   *Heather*

☐ If a misunderstanding can't be cleared up
immediately on the phone, it often bothers
me until the weekend.   *Agrimony, Star of Bethlehem*

☐ I try to cram into the weekends all the
things that people in normal relationships
can do throughout the week.   *Chicory, Vervain*

☐ I find my thoughts being more and more fixated
on the weekends and neglect my
other interests.   *Vervain, Heather, Red Chestnut, White Chestnut*

White Chestnut   Willow   Holly

Red Chestnut   Heather   Agrimony

Star of Bethlehem   Chicory   Vervain

22. I found out that my husband cheated on me.

"I always thought that Tom and I had a dream marriage. We have been married for fifteen years, and Tom has always reassured me about how happy he is with me. Then suddenly, at a company party, I heard that my husband has been having an affair with a colleague for a long time.

"My world fell apart. I can't understand it, because from my point of view we never had any problems. I did everything for him and fulfilled his every wish.

"Why did he do this to me? I don't deserve this. I will never forgive him for it! I'm deeply hurt and despairing. When I think of the future, I feel sick. All is lost, and I don't know how I can go on."

Recommendations

1. Write down your answers to the following question: "Which reactions and Flowers correspond to me?" If too few reactions are found, read the other cases in this chapter.
2. Refer as necessary to the reaction clusters section of this book.
3. Read the additional steps in the "How to Use This Book" chapter.

How do I react, and what Bach Flower patterns are identifiable?

☐ The news hit me like a ton of bricks.
I still feel stunned.   *Star of Bethlehem*

☐ I can't form clear thoughts;
the news keeps circling around
in my head.   *White Chestnut, Star of Bethlehem*

☐ I feel as if the rug has been pulled out from under
me and I'm about to fall into an abyss.   *Willow, Heather*

☐ I am deeply hurt and despairing.   *Holly, Sweet Chestnut*

☐ I feel betrayed and exploited. *Chicory, Willow*

☐ I am angry at myself for being so blind and
not realizing it. *Beech, Pine*

☐ I have no hope left that we will work
things out. *Sweet Chestnut, Gorse*

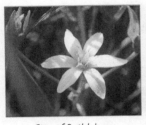

Star of Bethlehem

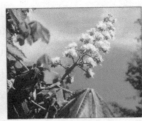

White Chestnut

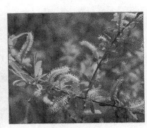

Willow

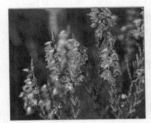

Heather

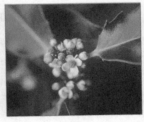

Holly

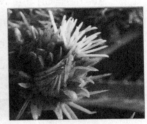

Sweet Chestnut

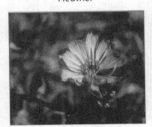

Chicory

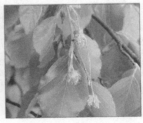

Beech

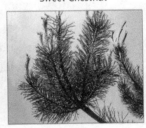

Pine

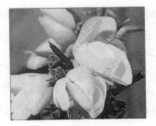

Gorse

23. My husband always accuses me of wasting money.

"Randy and I don't actually fight often, but when we do, it's always about money. My husband works for the planning commission, and we have a limited budget. We have two children (ages 5 and 7) and I'm trying to feed my family as healthfully as possible. But Randy can't understand my 'health kick.' He thinks products from the health food store are much too expensive.

"He accuses me of wasting money and would rather save every possible cent in our retirement account. 'That will take care of our future,' he always says. For me it's much more important for us to be well nourished, because I believe the best investment for the future is providing for one's health.

"At the moment we have very different views. I have often tried to talk with him about it, but with no success. These nerve-shattering arguments have gotten us nowhere, so I suggested that we go to a couple's counselor. But he doesn't want to spend the money."

Recommendations

1. Write down your answers to the following question: "Which reactions and Flowers correspond to me?" If too few reactions are found, read the other cases in this chapter.
2. Refer as necessary to the reaction clusters section of this book.
3. Read the additional steps in the "How to Use This Book" chapter.

How do I react, and what Bach Flower patterns are identifiable?

☐ I make so much effort to nourish my family properly,
but it isn't appreciated.   *Chicory*

☐ Since my husband is the one in our family who
earns the money, I feel dependent on him.   *Willow, Vine*

☐ The endless discussions wear me down,
because when we get to certain areas we
can't make any progress. *Chestnut Bud, Gorse*

☐ When we fight about money we become
mean and attack each other personally
in a way I never could have imagined. *Holly, Star of Bethlehem*

☐ I feel as though my husband doesn't understand
me and doesn't take me seriously. This makes me sad. *Mustard*

☐ The situation has gotten so bad for me that
I don't know what I can do anymore. *Sweet Chestnut*

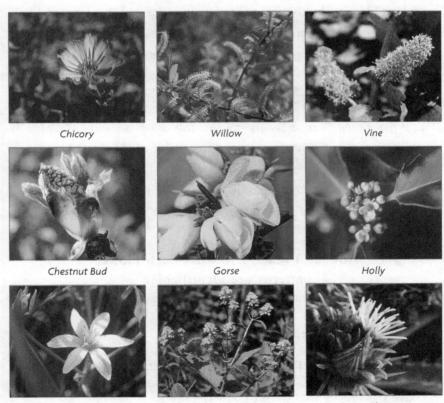

Chicory	*Willow*	*Vine*
Chestnut Bud	*Gorse*	*Holly*
Star of Bethlehem	*Mustard*	*Sweet Chestnut*

24. My husband is like an overgrown kid.

"I met Fred four years ago at a street festival, and I was impressed by his radiant charm and intelligence. When I learned that he was a high school teacher, I thought, 'This man must be very responsible, a good example to his students.'

"Only once we were married did I realize this was a mistaken conclusion. I am the only responsible one around here. For Fred, responsibility seems to be a nonexistent value. Of course he leaves it up to me to file our tax return. I also pay all the bills. I can't rely on him, even if he promises to pay them on time.

"Even in small things he shows a childish carelessness. For example, he likes to cook, but he leaves the kitchen looking like a battlefield. The more of his chores I take over, the more he pulls away from shared responsibility. I want a grown-up partner and not a big child."

Recommendations

1. Write down your answers to the following question: "Which reactions and Flowers correspond to me?" If too few reactions are found, read the other cases in this chapter.
2. Refer as necessary to the reaction clusters section of this book.
3. Read the additional steps in the "How to Use This Book" chapter.

How do I react, and what Bach Flower patterns are identifiable?

☐ I'm stressed from having to be responsible for everything.   *Elm*

☐ I am tired and drained.   *Olive, Elm*

☐ I feel alone because I can't rely on my partner.   *Heather, Willow*

☐ I have the feeling that if I let go of the reins, chaos would ensue.   *Cherry Plum, Elm*

☐ I think Fred is disorganized, superficial, and passive,
and I can hardly see any good sides to him anymore.   *Beech*

☐ Barely anything remains of my former feelings for him. *Holly, Gorse*

☐ I would love to change my husband,
but I don't know how.   *Chicory, Beech, Chestnut Bud*

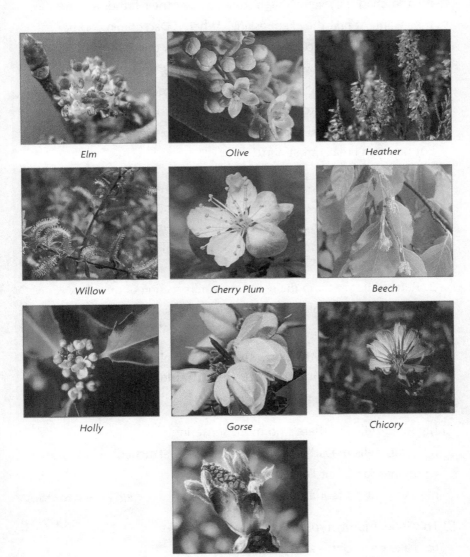

Elm

Olive

Heather

Willow

Cherry Plum

Beech

Holly

Gorse

Chicory

Chestnut Bud

25. Should I take my husband back?

"An event two years ago was the last straw in our ten-year marriage. I found out that Arthur was having an affair with his secretary. He moved to a different apartment and left me with Elizabeth (age 9) and Eric (age 7) in our townhouse. Of course the separation was hard for the children, even though they can see their father as often as they want. At first they kept asking, 'When is Dad coming home?'

"I tried to make up for the loss as much as possible and spent as much time as I could with them, even spending hours with Eric at the football field. I often wished my husband were back with me, but at the same time I was too proud to admit that to anyone.

"Now my husband wants to come back to me and the children, but how can I really trust him?"

Recommendations

1. Write down your answers to the following question: "Which reactions and Flowers correspond to me?" If too few reactions are found, read the other cases in this chapter.
2. Refer as necessary to the reaction clusters section of this book.
3. Read the additional steps in the "How to Use This Book" chapter.

How do I react, and what Bach Flower patterns are identifiable?

☐ I am uncertain what to do. I feel torn.   *Scleranthus*

☐ My mind tells me there's no more sense in it; my heart tells me otherwise. I still feel very attached to my husband, but I'm afraid he will betray me again, and I feel angry.   *Holly, Scleranthus*

☐ This indecision is typical for me. When I have to make decisions, I always doubt afterward whether they were right.   *Cerato, Scleranthus*

☐ If we don't get back together, I'm worried that I won't
be able to handle raising the children all by myself.   *Elm, Gentian*

☐ I always expect the maximum of myself. For this reason I
probably put too much strain on myself.   *Rock Water, Vervain*

☐ There is not much sense in asking advice from
others, because they can't help me.   *Water Violet*

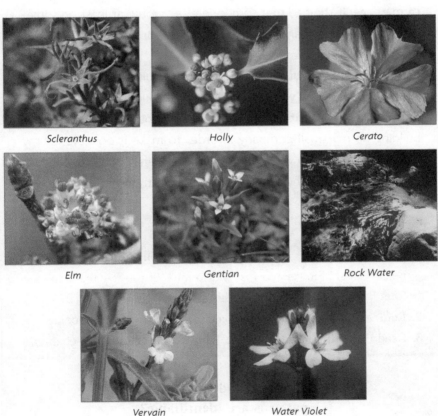

Scleranthus   Holly   Cerato

Elm   Gentian   Rock Water

Vervain   Water Violet

26. My wife has suddenly filed for divorce. Why?

"I have my own company, and, at age forty-two, I still look quite good, thanks to regular golf and tennis. I can hold conversations about all sorts of interesting things, and I generally consider myself a really nice, easygoing guy.

"So it totally threw me for a loop three months ago when Ingrid told me she had filed for divorce—out of the blue, after twelve years of marriage! If she had met someone else I would at least be somewhat able to understand her thought process. But why would she just give up everything like this?

"Then she moved out of our house pretty quickly, taking Mark (age 11) and Anna (8) along with her. I can't stop thinking about her accusation that I am insensitive and egotistical. I've put a lot of work into building up my small company in order to make it possible for my family to live the way we do. Now I am completely at a loss, because I don't know what I should have done differently."

Recommendations

1. Write down your answers to the following question: "Which reactions and Flowers correspond to me?" If too few reactions are found, read the other cases in this chapter.
2. Refer as necessary to the reaction clusters section of this book.
3. Read the additional steps in the "How to Use This Book" chapter.

How do I react, and what Bach Flower patterns are identifiable?

☐ I am at a complete loss and keep
questioning myself.   *Cerato, Beech*

☐ My pride is injured. I am deeply hurt.   *Holly, Willow*

☐ My thoughts keep circling around what I might
have done wrong.   *White Chestnut*

☐ Right away, I began to have an affair with
an old girlfriend. She makes me feel like I'm
still a worthwhile man.   *Wild Oat, Larch, Vervain*

☐ I'm secretly afraid to commit to a new woman
because I might not be able to meet
her expectations.   *Larch, Gentian*

☐ I'm afraid that my children will be alienated from me.   *Mimulus*

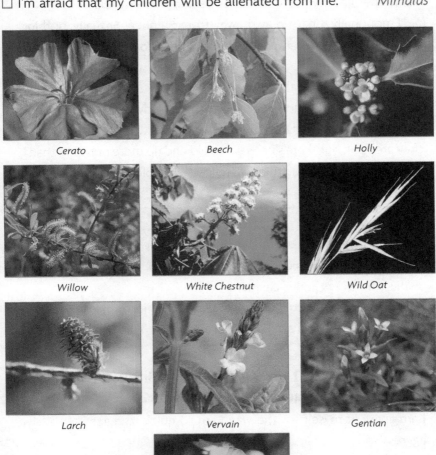

Cerato · Beech · Holly

Willow · White Chestnut · Wild Oat

Larch · Vervain · Gentian

Mimulus

27. We've gotten tired of each other, but I'm scared of the separation.

"After ten years of marriage, our relationship is continuing by force of habit, and I don't believe it can change now. When we talk with each other, an aggressive tone immediately takes over, and we do nothing but fight. Outwardly we have a harmonious marriage. Only a few of our friends know what actually lies behind that exterior.

"Emotionally, I have drawn away from Stephen. Sexually, nothing has happened between us for a long time. I don't want to keep on living this lie, but I'm scared of the separation: scared of being alone and scared of making the wrong decision.

"My friends who know about the situation advise me against separating. They say, 'You'll never find such a good partner again!' Perhaps they are right, but there's no way I could end up more unhappy than I currently am. I keep torturing myself with terrible doubts."

Recommendations

1. Write down your answers to the following question: Which reactions and Flowers correspond to me? If too few reactions are found, read the other cases in this chapter.
2. Refer as necessary to the reaction clusters section of this book.
3. Read the additional steps in the "How to Use This Book" chapter.

How do I react, and what Bach Flower patterns are identifiable?

☐ I am angry at myself for the way I am so quick to react aggressively.   *Holly*

☐ I won't let on how inwardly torn I am, because I don't want people to gossip about us.   *Agrimony*

☐ I am afraid of hurting my husband when I tell him
I don't love him anymore. *Pine, Mimulus*

☐ It's no simple matter to give up everything
after ten years of marriage. The idea
makes me sad. *Honeysuckle, Mustard*

☐ I'm scared of making the wrong decision. *Mimulus, Scleranthus*

☐ When I compare my marriage with the relationships
my girlfriends are in, I feel like a failure. *Larch*

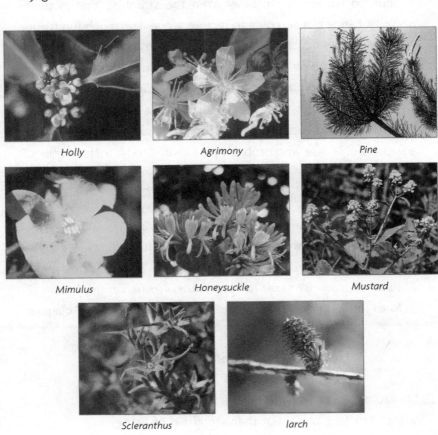

Holly   *Agrimony*   *Pine*

Mimulus   *Honeysuckle*   *Mustard*

Scleranthus   *larch*

28. Thirty-something and single: When I don't have anything going on over the weekend, I feel emotionally lost.

"I am single. Not by choice, but just because things have turned out that way. I was always waiting for some big Hollywood romance, but my 'dream partner' hasn't shown up yet. I'm fine with my single status from Monday to Friday. As a lawyer in a joint practice, I feel like an important part of a functioning society, and I know that my work is meaningful. As I said, from Monday to Friday.

"But on weekends I'm away from the structure that gives me security. Eating out or going to movies alone isn't much fun for me, because there's no one I can talk to. I only visit my sister once in a while so as not to be constantly confronted with her happy family.

"I also dread holidays. New Year's Eve is approaching and I haven't been invited to anything. I feel uncomfortable about inviting myself over to my friends' places, because I assume that everyone sees me as a successful lawyer who probably gets invited to all sorts of things."

Recommendations

1. Write down your answers to the following question: "Which reactions and Flowers correspond to me?" If too few reactions are found, read the other cases in this chapter.
2. Refer as necessary to the reaction clusters section of this book.
3. Read the additional steps in the "How to Use This Book" chapter.

How do I react, and what Bach Flower patterns are identifiable?

☐ Sometimes I just want to let the weekend come along without making plans, but then I'm afraid of being alone and feeling lonely and unwanted.   *Mimulus, Heather*

☐ I'm jealous of my sister's happy family life.   *Holly*

☐ I actually yearn for a steady partner,
  but I can't commit.   *Agrimony, Water Violet*

☐ I can't enjoy a relaxing weekend alone, even
  though it would do me good.   *Rock Water*

☐ I'm afraid of getting on other people's nerves when I call
  to plan something with them for the weekend.
  I don't want to let down my guard and admit,
  for example, that I haven't been invited
  anywhere for New Year's Eve.   *Water Violet, Agrimony*

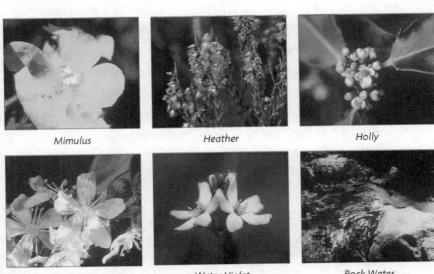

Mimulus   Heather   Holly

Agrimony   Water Violet   Rock Water

29. My friend sees me as nothing but a psychic dumping ground.

"Sally and I met three years ago in a painting class and immediately empathized with one another. We are almost the same age—early forties—both single, and have many interests in common. We go on vacations together and meet up almost every weekend.

"I like Sally a lot, but there's one thing that has always annoyed me about her: she unloads all her job stress and worries about her sick mother on me. She talks about these things for hours on end.

"I've always had an open ear for her, even though sometimes she has called me in the middle of the night. But when I try to talk with her about any of my own problems, she always interrupts and shifts the subject over to one of her experiences. My story then becomes her story. She doesn't listen to me at all anymore, and I've given up trying to talk to her about things that happen in my life.

"I wonder if I'm really just her psychic dumping ground. This is putting a burden on our friendship. Actually I need to talk to her about it, but I'm afraid to bring it up."

Recommendations

1. Write down your answers to the following question: "Which reactions and Flowers correspond to me?" If too few reactions are found, read the other cases in this chapter.
2. Refer as necessary to the reaction clusters section of this book.
3. Read the additional steps in the "How to Use This Book" chapter.

How do I react, and what Bach Flower patterns are identifiable?

☐ I can't hold my own against my friend's
torrent of words.   *Centaury*

☐ I have the feeling that my problems don't matter to her.
Sometimes I believe that for her, I'm just the
means to an end. *Gentian, Holly*

☐ I often feel hurt, but so far I've always put a
good face on things. *Holly, Agrimony*

☐ I'm afraid to criticize my friend, for fear of losing
our friendship. *Chicory, Mimulus*

☐ If we were no longer friends, I would be
completely lost. *Heather, Red Chestnut*

☐ I'm afraid of having to spend my free time
alone again. *Mimulus*

Centaury

Gentian

Holly

Agrimony

Chicory

Mimulus

Heather

Red Chestnut

30. I've moved my bedridden mother in with me.

"My mother (age 87) has been bedridden and senile for two years. I took her in because I wanted to give her back all the love and care that she once gave to me. Also, I am single, retired, and have a spare room. My brother isn't in a position to take in our mother because he has his own family.

"Now I take care of my mother with the help of a hired nurse, but even with that, the situation is quite difficult. Whenever I go out, whether to the movies, the gym, or to meet friends, I can't fully enjoy it. It is also very problematic to organize vacations. I have to think constantly about what's going on at home and worry whether my mother is being cared for properly.

"Since taking her in, my life has changed completely. It's wearing me down, both psychically and physically, much more than I would have imagined. So for a while now I've been wrestling with the decision of whether to put my mother in a nursing home."

Recommendations

1. Write down your answers to the following question: "Which reactions and Flowers correspond to me?" If too few reactions are found, read the other cases in this chapter.
2. Refer as necessary to the reaction clusters section of this book.
3. Read the additional steps in the "How to Use This Book" chapter.

How do I react, and what Bach Flower patterns are identifiable?

☐ I am completely worn out and I feel like
a martyr, silently carrying this burden
day after day.   *Olive, Hornbeam, Oak*

☐ I feel disappointed that no one in my family
realizes what I go through every day.   *Chicory, Gentian*

☐ I am secretly angry at my brother for
leaving so much of the work to me. *Agrimony, Holly, Willow*

☐ I can't fully enjoy my few free-time activities
because my thoughts are always with my mother. *Red Chestnut*

☐ Sometimes I even wish my mother would pass
away soon, but then I berate myself bitterly for
having such thoughts. *Pine*

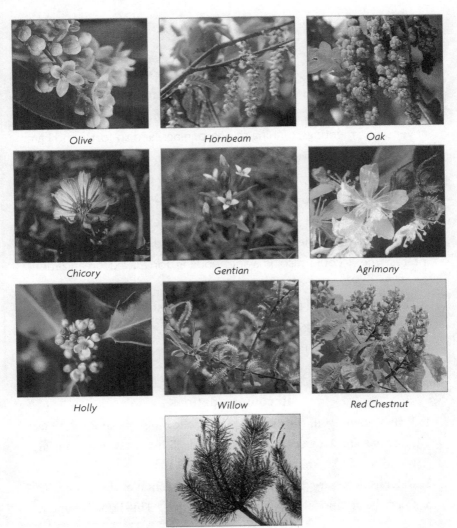

Olive

Hornbeam

Oak

Chicory

Gentian

Agrimony

Holly

Willow

Red Chestnut

Pine

Career and Professional Life

31. Help, I'm in the wrong job!

"I am thirty-five years old and a local reporter for a small newspaper. To be honest, the job is simply not fulfilling. I'm always being sent to cover union meetings, tanning salon openings, and so forth, and I am never done with work before 9:00 p.m. It was my dream to become a journalist, but the day-to-day reality is entirely different.

"I'm depressed and worn out and would like to change my professional direction. As a freelance journalist, for example, I would have many more possibilities, including being able to report on things that interest me. I could also imagine working for an aid organization, where at least my work would be for a good cause.

"But my boyfriend and my family are earnestly advising me not to quit my job. I'm torn: Should I hold on to my security, or take the risk and listen to my inner voice?"

Recommendations

1. Write down your answers to the following question: "Which reactions and Flowers correspond to me?" If too few reactions are found, read the other cases in this chapter.
2. Refer as necessary to the reaction clusters section of this book.
3. Read the additional steps in the "How to Use This Book" chapter.

How do I react, and what Bach Flower patterns are identifiable?

☐ It is taking more and more energy each morning to drag myself to the office. *Hornbeam*

☐ My thoughts are continually revolving around the subject of my profession. Sometimes I lie awake half the night thinking and thinking about it. *White Chestnut*

☐ I vacillate between wanting security and imagining the possibility of finally doing what fulfills me and gets me further in life. *Scleranthus*

☐ New and tempting career ideas keep occurring to me, but there is no common theme to them. *Clematis, Wild Oat*

☐ It makes me unsure when everyone I know advises me not to change things. *Walnut*

☐ Right now I cannot access my own intuition, which I've always relied upon in the past for making important decisions. *Cerato*

Hornbeam

White Chestnut

Scleranthus

Clematis

Wild Oat

Walnut

Cerato

32. I'm scared of public speaking.

"I am a doctor in a psychiatric clinic. In our department we've developed a therapy project that is slated to be presented to a panel of our colleagues. Since I led the project, the head doctor thinks I should also present it. His intention is to give me an opportunity to distinguish myself. I'm very grateful to him for this, but at the same time I'm very anxious about this presentation.

"All my life I've been incapable of public speaking. The very first time I had to give a presentation in school, I blushed, began stuttering, and couldn't remember anything. Somehow I was able to get by okay in school, but in classes I avoided such situations at all costs.

"Now I feel that if I want to have a career, I can't avoid having to speak in public sometimes. Even though I know I can read from a sheet of paper and the team has prepared a Power Point display for me, I still break out in a cold sweat when I think about the lecture date."

Recommendations

1. Write down your answers to the following question: "Which reactions and Flowers correspond to me?" If too few reactions are found, read the other cases in this chapter.
2. Refer as necessary to the reaction clusters section of this book.
3. Read the additional steps in the "How to Use This Book" chapter.

How do I react, and what Bach Flower patterns are identifiable?

☐ When I think about the lecture I get so nervous that my heart jumps into my throat and all the blood rushes to my head.   *Rock Rose*

☐ When I imagine myself standing up there and turning all red, I feel like a helpless victim.   *Willow, Rock Rose*

☐ I know my fear is unreasonable. I'm trying to
keep from showing the stage fright I'm already feeling. *Agrimony*

☐ I am already picturing all the things that could go wrong. *Gentian*

☐ I put great pressure on myself because I want
everything to be perfect. *Vervain*

☐ I'm sure my coworkers on the team are better
suited for this task than I am. *Larch*

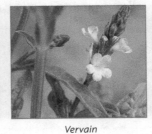

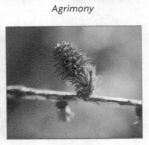

Rock Rose *Willow* *Agrimony*

Gentian *Vervain* *Larch*

33. I always take on more responsibilities than I can comfortably handle.

"Recently I lost my steady job as a translator and became a freelancer. I get some work from my former employer from time to time, but I can't live on that alone. So I'm forced to take on projects from translation agencies.

"This puts me under increasing pressure, because I don't want to disappoint my clients. The work is piling up on my desk because I've promised to deliver the translations in a few days' time. I almost always take on too many projects at once, and often fall behind.

"Then I feel like I'm drowning in my work, so I translate deep into the night and on the weekends. Even on vacations I take my laptop with me, and my personal life is nonexistent. I can't plan anything, I eat only fast food, and I don't sleep enough. I can't go on like this!"

Recommendations

1. Write down your answers to the following question: "Which reactions and Flowers correspond to me?" If too few reactions are found, read the other cases in this chapter.
2. Refer as necessary to the reaction clusters section of this book.
3. Read the additional steps in the "How to Use This Book" chapter.

How do I react, and what Bach Flower patterns are identifiable?

☐ I feel like I'm drowning in my work; I'm totally
overwhelmed. *Willow, Rock Rose*

☐ I reproach myself for not organizing myself
better as an independent worker. *Larch, Elm, Pine*

☐ I don't want to turn down any work and
possibly lose clients. *Mimulus, Centaury*

☐ There are days I'd rather just stay in bed,
and I wish I had some elves to do
the work for me.   *Clematis, Hornbeam, Star of Bethlehem*

☐ Other people tell me these are normal start-up
challenges and I should learn to adjust my
deadlines to meet my own needs.   *Centaury, Vine, Elm*

☐ I feel like a hamster on a wheel, running in
place while my life slips past me.   *Oak, Impatiens*

Willow

Rock Rose

Larch

Elm

Pine

Mimulus

Centaury

Clematis

Hornbeam

Star of Bethlehem

Vine

Oak

Impatiens

34. I've suddenly been promoted to management, but I'm not equal to the role.

"While working as an electrical engineer for a big car manufacturing company, I recently got the chance to take over a leading position. Suddenly I have more than twenty workers under me. But I'm having a hard time adjusting to my new role as manager and leader.

"I used to be able to concentrate on my technical work as a specialist, but these abilities hardly come into play anymore. Instead I am constantly pressured by demands from all sides. Upper management sets tight deadlines for my department, but the workers have made it clear that they can't meet those deadlines without loss of quality.

"I keep having to throw out my plans and create new ones in order to be fair to all parties. Sometimes I would rather give up my management title and salary just to get back my peace of mind."

Recommendations

1. Write down your answers to the following question: "Which reactions and Flowers correspond to me? If too few reactions are found, read the other cases in this chapter."
2. Refer as necessary to the reaction clusters section of this book.
3. Read the additional steps in the "How to Use This Book" chapter.

How do I react, and what Bach Flower patterns are identifiable?

☐ It's difficult for me to step out of my role as a specialist and keep the larger perspective of the whole company in mind when I make decisions.   *Crab Apple*

☐ I have to live with the fact that my coworkers, for whom I'm responsible, will make mistakes.   *Elm*

☐ My coworkers expect me to pass along their complaints to those

in charge. But often I have inhibitions about presenting these
concerns to upper management. *Centaury, Mimulus*

☐ It's difficult for me to require my colleagues to accept
my decisions without discussion in certain cases. *Vine, Mimulus*

☐ In my vulnerable role I often feel lonely and
shut out, because camaraderie with my coworkers
is no longer possible. *Heather, Willow*

☐ Sometimes I wish I had my old position
back, where I wasn't confronted with so
many problems every day. *Water Violet, Honeysuckle*

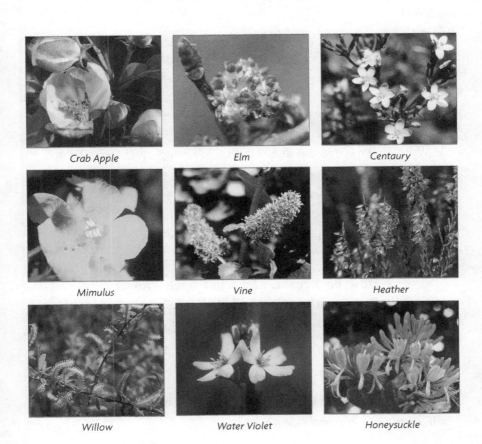

Crab Apple   Elm   Centaury

Mimulus   Vine   Heather

Willow   Water Violet   Honeysuckle

35. I feel as if I'm being attacked.

"I am fifty-two years old, and for more than thirty years I've been working as an administrator for my company. About a year ago I got a new boss, for whom I can do absolutely nothing right. He criticizes my appearance, my clothing, my haircut, and—even worse—my work performance. He accuses me of not working precisely enough and being too slow. My old boss never said anything like that to me!

"My husband has advised me to simply ignore these accusations. He's even implied that there must be something to them, considering that my boss repeats them constantly. He says I shouldn't compromise my job but instead try to improve in the areas my new boss criticizes.

"I wonder whether I should listen to my husband or go to workers' arbitration, because I've seen my new boss pestering other women my age as well."

Recommendations

1. Write down your answers to the following question: "Which reactions and Flowers correspond to me?" If too few reactions are found, read the other cases in this chapter.
2. Refer as necessary to the reaction clusters section of this book.
3. Read the additional steps in the "How to Use This Book" chapter.

How do I react, and what Bach Flower patterns are identifiable?

☐ I am completely uncertain and don't know what to do. I don't know whether my husband's advice is correct or not.   *Cerato*

☐ I am doubting myself as a person, and my feeling of self-worth is completely destroyed.   *Larch*

☐ There are days when I feel sick from worry
in the morning, and I would much rather not
go to work.   *Rock Rose, Willow*

☐ In the office I always feel on edge, wondering
what will go wrong next.   *Cherry Plum, Rock Rose*

☐ I'm totally intimidated, and I hardly trust
myself even to speak privately with my colleagues
or go out for coffee with them.   *Mimulus*

☐ I lie awake at night and worry about the things
I'll have to face the next morning.   *White Chestnut, Aspen*

Cerato   Larch   Rock Rose

Willow   Cherry Plum   Mimulus

White Chestnut   Aspen

36. I feel burned out.

"I've been working for fifteen years as a department manager in a photo shop. I'm fifty-three years old and feel completely tired and burned out. Although I really like my profession and overall I've been highly engaged in it—always the first to arrive in the morning and the last to leave at night—now I can barely summon the energy to go to work.

"I used to have a keen interest in every technical detail. Lately there have been rapid new developments in the field of photography, but I have no more interest in keeping up with them. I'd rather leave it to my coworkers.

"I feel more and more like a stranger in my own territory. I don't feel things anymore; I just function mechanically like a robot. I don't know how much longer I can stand this. I'm trying to keep my situation hidden from my family. I'm able to do this to a great extent, but I'm still very depressed."

Recommendations

1. Write down your answers to the following question: "Which reactions and Flowers correspond to me?" If too few reactions are found, read the other cases in this chapter.
2. Refer as necessary to the reaction clusters section of this book.
3. Read the additional steps in the "How to Use This Book" chapter.

How do I react, and what Bach Flower patterns are identifiable?

☐ I have no more energy, no more drive,
no motivation to go to work. *Olive, Hornbeam, Wild Rose*

☐ I have become very thin-skinned, and I often
feel irritable and aggressive. *Star of Bethlehem, Holly, Impatiens*

☐ I have withdrawn into myself because social contact overwhelms me. I also don't have any more interest in physical activity. *Water Violet, Mustard*

☐ My thoughts always revolve around negative things, and I can't grab onto anything positive anymore. *White Chestnut, Gentian*

☐ I am totally depressed and feel like a useless failure who no longer has a grip on life. *Larch, Pine, Mustard*

☐ I would most like to run away and leave it all behind. *Sweet Chestnut, Clematis*

Olive

Hornbeam

Wild Rose

Star of Bethlehem

Holly

Impatiens

Water Violet

Mustard

White Chestnut

Gentian

Larch

Pine

Sweet Chestnut

Clematis

37. I've lost my job, and I have massive fear and anxiety.

"About six months ago, at the age of forty-eight, I was let go from my job as manager in a printing company. I can see my employer's point of view, because business has dropped dramatically and they have to cut costs. But getting laid off was a shock to me.

"I worked for this company for twenty years, and in some way I felt proprietary about it—it was my life. Since then I have been plagued by massive fear and anxiety. I've applied to countless other jobs but received nothing but rejection. I always thought my good connections would be helpful to me, but most people are afraid for their jobs. It is all so much more difficult than I anticipated.

"Now I'm afraid of not finding any work at all. I have a huge amount of debt, a house, and a family with three children, two of them still in school. For the moment I am still financially secure, but what if I have to go on welfare? What a nightmare!"

Recommendations

1. Write down your answers to the following question: "Which reactions and Flowers correspond to me?" If too few reactions are found, read the other cases in this chapter.
2. Refer as necessary to the reaction clusters section of this book.
3. Read the additional steps in the "How to Use This Book" chapter.

How do I react, and what Bach Flower patterns are identifiable?

☐ I still can't believe that I was actually dismissed
from my job. *Star of Bethlehem*

☐ I can't imagine starting a new type of
career now. *Wild Oat, Chestnut Bud*

☐ I always worked hard and people were satisfied with my
performance. Now I'm wondering what I did wrong. *Larch*

☐ Every day I miss my desk, my coworkers,
   the meetings, even the pressure of deadlines.   *Honeysuckle*

☐ I often lie awake at night and picture what it will be like when
   we no longer have a roof over our heads, no longer
   own a car, and my wife and I have to make money
   by cleaning houses.   *Rock Rose, Aspen, White Chestnut*

☐ Despite all my efforts to find a new job, I'm
   beginning to feel deeply certain that I'll
   never find one.   *Vervain, Wild Rose*

☐ Although I don't show it to my family,
   I'm angry at myself for having disappointed
   them so bitterly.   *Pine, Gentian*

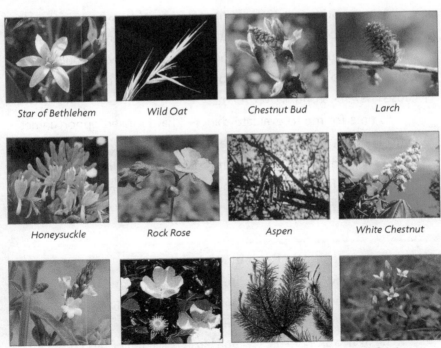

Star of Bethlehem   *Wild Oat*   *Chestnut Bud*   *Larch*

Honeysuckle   *Rock Rose*   *Aspen*   *White Chestnut*

Vervain   *Wild Rose*   *Pine*   *Gentian*

Aging

38. I'm upset about getting older.

"I'm forty-eight years old. Recently a young man gave up his seat to me on the bus. That was when I suddenly realized that I had gotten old. I had always suppressed the idea, but now I'm aware that my life isn't ahead of me anymore. I feel as if the time has come to get used to that fact, and this is a problem for me.

"Many questions are tormenting me: As an older woman, am I less interesting socially? Am I still at all attractive to men? Should I stop buying youthful clothes even though they still fit me? Should I take hormone supplements? My menopausal difficulties unsettle me because I have no control over them.

"It's time for me to evaluate things—I have missed opportunities in my life that are no longer available to me. I envy the many opportunities for growth that my children still have. My girlfriend tells me that a wonderful time of life is now ahead of me, but at the moment I can't believe that at all."

Recommendations

1. Write down your answers to the following question: "Which reactions and Flowers correspond to me?" If too few reactions are found, read the other cases in this chapter.
2. Refer as necessary to the reaction clusters section of this book.
3. Read the additional steps in the "How to Use This Book" chapter.

How do I react, and what Bach Flower patterns are identifiable?

☐ I catch myself going through the exact same mood swings
my mother used to experience. Now I understand.   *Honeysuckle*

☐ I am more sensitive and easily hurt than I
was in previous years.   *Star of Bethlehem, Holly*

☐ I envy my daughter's good looks and vitality.   *Holly*

☐ I catch myself thinking: "I can't do that anymore,
not at my age."   *Gorse*

☐ I'm afraid of this new phase of life.   *Mimulus, Walnut*

☐ I am often subject to mood swings, and often overwhelmed by sadness, without any reason.   *Scleranthus, Mustard*

Honeysuckle

Star of Bethlehem

Holly

Gorse

Mimulus

Walnut

Scleranthus

Mustard

39. I'm having trouble adjusting to my husband's retirement.

"My husband was successfully engaged in foreign business, so he often spent days at a time away from home. This was a good arrangement for me, allowing me to fill my time in pursuing many different interests. Since he retired, he is home almost twenty-four hours a day.

"This is a huge change for me. It begins with the morning paper—I used to have it all to myself; now he wants to read it at the same time as I do. He gets in my way around the house, but then he spends hours driving around on his Harley, something he dreamed about for years.

"I'm discovering completely unknown sides of him, sides I don't like and wish he would change. But he doesn't think about it. More and more conflicts are emerging between our daily life and his various rituals, so our everyday life needs to be completely restructured.

"We had made plans together for what to do during our retirement, but now my husband suddenly has his own, new life—without me. How can we get our diverging paths back onto a single track?"

Recommendations

1. Write down your answers to the following question: "Which reactions and Flowers correspond to me?" If too few reactions are found, read the other cases in this chapter.
2. Refer as necessary to the reaction clusters section of this book.
3. Read the additional steps in the "How to Use This Book" chapter.

How do I react, and what Bach Flower patterns are identifiable?

☐ I feel like I'm not free anymore; instead I'm
restricted, watched, and controlled.   *Cherry Plum, Vine*

☐ It makes me angry that I share so much with my husband
and often have to arrange things with him.   *Holly*

☐ Since he does so many things by himself now, I feel betrayed,
neglected, and useless.   *Heather, Willow*

☐ I become impatient quickly, and I'm growing
increasingly intolerant.   *Impatiens, Beech*

☐ I also have a bad conscience; I feel awful.   *Pine*

☐ On the other hand, my reactions seem so absurd
and childish to me. I'm ashamed of my behavior,
because really I'm good-natured and easygoing.   *Beech, Larch*

☐ We have to find a new pattern for daily life,
but it's hard for me to give up my familiar habits.   *Walnut*

☐ I can't imagine what this new life is going to be like.   *Wild Oat*

Cherry Plum

Vine

Holly

Heather

Willow

Impatiens

Beech

Larch

Walnut

Pine

Wild Oat

40. Now that I'm retired, I feel useless and frustrated.

"I recently retired. I was really looking forward to it: no more rat race, sleeping as long as I please, and doing only whatever I enjoy. Now I do all that, but I'm not happy. This 'idyllic time' is nothing like what I had imagined.

"When I try to help out around the house, they just tell me not to get in the way since I'll do it all wrong anyway. I feel like a stranger in my own house. My family is pressuring me to find a hobby, but I have no real idea what I'd like to do.

"Most of my friends are still working, so I see much less of them and don't feel like I'm really one of them. Sometimes I wish I could turn back time, because I don't know how I can get out of this frustrating limbo. The idea that the rest of my life will be like this terrifies me."

Recommendations

1. Write down your answers to the following question: "Which reactions and Flowers correspond to me?" If too few reactions are found, read the other cases in this chapter.
2. Refer as necessary to the reaction clusters section of this book.
3. Read the additional steps in the "How to Use This Book" chapter.

How do I react, and what Bach Flower patterns are identifiable?

☐ I am disappointed by my retirement.   *Gentian*

☐ I don't know what to do with my life anymore.   *Wild Oat*

☐ I feel incapable and superfluous.   *Larch*

☐ I could just about fly off the handle. I'm very
angry because I don't know how I can change
my situation. *Cherry Plum, Holly*

☐ Even though I now have time to sleep
late, I always wake up at 6:00 a.m.
So I try to make myself stay in
bed until 8:00. *Chestnut Bud, Rock Water*

☐ I often yearn to have my working days back. *Honeysuckle*

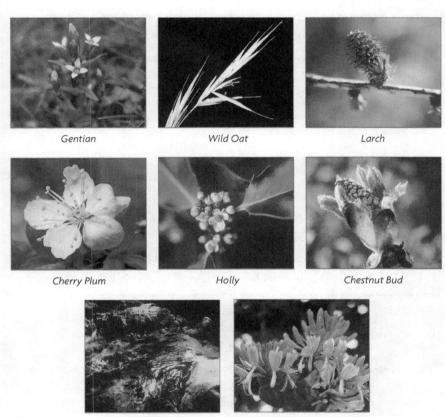

Gentian   Wild Oat   Larch

Cherry Plum   Holly   Chestnut Bud

Rock Water   Honeysuckle

41. I feel exploited in my role as a grandmother.

"I work from home as a children's book editor, but my family is at least as important to me as my profession. This puts me in a quandary. My two grown-up sons are always stopping by unannounced with their wives and children, and they expect me, as the grandmother, to be constantly available to them.

"Sometimes the two young families seem to consume me completely. They leave me very little free space, and they are infringing on my private life. I suppress my anger and don't set boundaries for them. Sometimes I wonder if I let all this happen to me just because I want to keep feeling needed.

"Now the situation has come to a head. In a week I have to submit a manuscript to my publisher, but my daughter-in-law is expecting me to take care of two of my grandchildren while she goes to a weekend seminar with my son."

Recommendations

1. Write down your answers to the following question: "Which reactions and Flowers correspond to me?" If too few reactions are found, read the other cases in this chapter.
2. Refer as necessary to the reaction clusters section of this book.
3. Read the additional steps in the "How to Use This Book" chapter.

How do I react, and what Bach Flower patterns are identifiable?

☐ Although I'm happy about all this close family contact, I feel over-whelmed by it.   *Scleranthus, Rock Rose*

☐ I am suppressing my anger and holding myself back from stating my own needs clearly.   *Cherry Plum, Centaury*

☐ I give my family a great deal of my time and energy, but I don't get enough in return.   *Chicory, Olive*

☐ I'm disappointed that my family doesn't acknowledge that I have my own life or take my profession seriously. *Gentian, Willow*

☐ Sometimes I get so angry that I call up my friend on the phone and whine. *Rock Rose, Mustard*

☐ I have the feeling that because I am still so closely involved in my sons' lives their well-being is a little too important to me. *Red Chestnut*

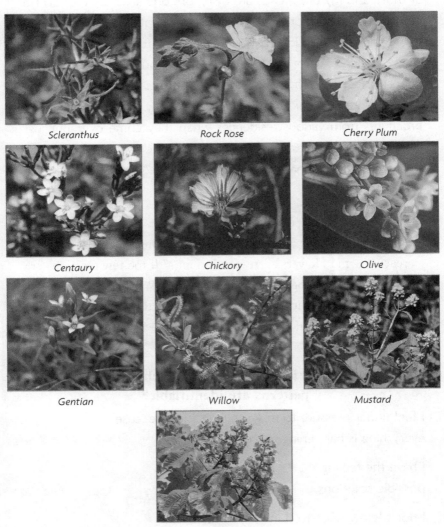

Scleranthus

Rock Rose

Cherry Plum

Centaury

Chickory

Olive

Gentian

Willow

Mustard

Red Chestnut

42. The idea of having to move into a senior home makes me panic.

"Seven years after my husband's death, I'm still living by myself in our single-family home. At eighty-two I am still mentally on the ball, but getting up and down the stairs is becoming more difficult.

"My children and grandchildren visit me every two or three weeks at most, and my old friends are dying off, one after another, so I'm getting more and more lonely. Sometimes I catch myself talking to myself, since I often don't have anyone to talk to for days at a time.

"My children, unfortunately, don't have enough room to take me in. I can understand that. They're advising me more and more urgently to move into a senior home, and recently they've been bringing me brochures from various residences when they come over. But just looking at them makes me panic, because I never want to move to an old folks' home, no matter how ritzy it may be."

Recommendations

1. Write down your answers to the following question: "Which reactions and Flowers correspond to me?" If too few reactions are found, read the other cases in this chapter.
2. Refer as necessary to the reaction clusters section of this book.
3. Read the additional steps in the "How to Use This Book" chapter.

How do I react, and what Bach Flower patterns are identifiable?

☐ I feel under pressure to make this decision because
everything is happening too quickly for me.   *Cherry Plum, Vine*

☐ I have the feeling that there may be other
possible solutions.   *Aspen, Wild Oat*

☐ I don't know what to think anymore, or
whom to ask for advice.   *Cerato*

☐ If I move into a senior home, I know for sure that it marks
the end stage of my life. This depresses me. *Mustard, Gentian*

☐ The thought of giving up all the beloved things
around me, connected with so many memories,
makes me panic. *Honeysuckle, Rock Rose*

☐ When I picture a senior home in my mind, I see endless
corridors and dismal rooms, like a vast hospital. *Clematis, Gentian*

☐ I'm afraid of becoming so senile that someone
else will have to make my decisions for me. *Mimulus, Aspen, Vine*

Cherry Plum

Vine

Aspen

Wild Oat

Cerato

Mustard

Gentian

Honeysuckle

Rock Rose

Clematis

Mimulus

Other Crises

43. My nineteen-year-old son died suddenly.

"It's been seven months now, but I still haven't assimilated it. They found Mike at the bottom of the cliff he'd driven off in the new car we'd given him for graduation. The only comfort for us—if it's possible to speak of comfort in this kind of situation—is that he probably died instantly.

"Now I am afraid of losing my wife as well, because the different ways in which we are dealing with the loss are drawing us further and further apart. Our marriage is threatening to disintegrate, not least because Doris doesn't want to sleep with me anymore. She keeps going to various clairvoyants who claim to be able to establish contact with the dead, and she's getting more and more crazy.

"Meanwhile, I'm taking every opportunity to work overtime, and I'm drinking more than is good for me at the pub I own—all in an effort to spend as little time as possible in our sad house."

Recommendations

1. Write down your answers to the following question: "Which reactions and Flowers correspond to me?" If too few reactions are found, read the other cases in this chapter.
2. Refer as necessary to the reaction clusters section of this book.
3. Read the additional steps in the "How to Use This Book" chapter.

How do I react, and what Bach Flower patterns are identifiable?

☐ I feel awful for having given our son the new car in
which he crashed. *Pine*

☐ I can't mope around at work in the pub. But I also
can't act as if nothing has happened. *Cerato, Agrimony*

☐ Sometimes I would rather not come home at all. All I
see there is tear-stained faces. *Agrimony, Water Violet, Mimulus*

☐ In my sadness, I feel physically repelled from my wife. *Larch, Willow*

☐ I completely reject this esoteric stuff my wife is pursuing.
It's not a solution. *Beech*

☐ Our son was supposed to take over the pub one day, while I drew
away from it little by little. I am upset that after this bitter end, I
have to continue working more than I'd like. *Willow, Honeysuckle*

Pine

Cerato

Agrimony

Water Violet

Mimulus

Larch

Willow

Beech

Honeysuckle

44. Since my accident, I can't sleep anymore.

"Recently, driving my car back from my Italian class in the evening, I didn't see a cyclist riding across a crosswalk. My car bumper hit the young woman's bike wheel, and she was thrown into the street. I immediately stopped and ran over to help her. She groaned and said her arm hurt.

"I called the police on my cell phone, and the ambulance came as well. It turned out that her arm was broken. Of course I came to the hospital the next day and brought her flowers and apologized, but the shock is still with me. Every night I see that moment when my car hit the bike wheel, as if in a slow-motion loop. I can't get the images out of my head."

Recommendations

1. Write down your answers to the following question: "Which reactions and Flowers correspond to me?" If too few reactions are found, read the other cases in this chapter.
2. Refer as necessary to the reaction clusters section of this book.
3. Read the additional steps in the "How to Use This Book" chapter.

How do I react, and what Bach Flower patterns are identifiable?

☐ This event was a huge shock for me.   *Star of Bethlehem*

☐ My heart races and I can hardly eat.   *Rock Rose*

☐ I keep agonizing over how I could have avoided
this accident by acting just a second sooner.   *White Chestnut*

☐ Despite having apologized and brought her
flowers, I still feel deeply guilty.   *Pine*

☐ I simply can't forgive myself for causing another
person so much pain through just a moment
of inattentiveness. *Rock Water, Beech*

☐ I can't get the images of the accident out
of my head. *Honeysuckle*

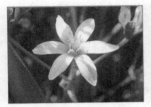
Star of Bethlehem

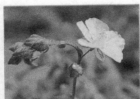
Rock Rose

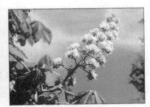
White Chestnut

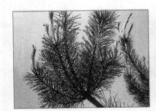
Pine

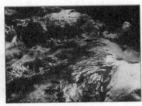
Rock Water

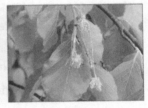
Beech

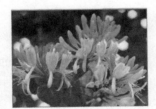
Honeysuckle

45. As a foreigner, I keep going back and forth on whether I should stay in the United States.

"I moved to the United States from India thirty years ago with my family because of a good job offer. At the time the move seemed like a good decision, and I have climbed several steps up the career ladder. The last step, though, remains out of reach for me, even though I have the job requirements.

"I have the feeling that it's because I'm a foreigner. Or because, although I speak English fluently, I don't have the same way with words that I do in my native language, in which I can be very funny and entertaining. Also, a couple of weeks ago, I was openly insulted on the street because of my skin color.

"Recently I've noticed myself listening to more sitar music and going to more Indian stores than I did in the past. More and more I feel homesick as I never did before. All this makes me wonder whether I really want to spend my twilight years in the United States or if I would rather go back to my homeland."

Recommendations

1. Write down your answers to the following question: "Which reactions and Flowers correspond to me?" If too few reactions are found, read the other cases in this chapter.
2. Refer as necessary to the reaction clusters section of this book.
3. Read the additional steps in the "How to Use This Book" chapter.

How do I react, and what Bach Flower patterns are identifiable?

☐ Sometimes I feel like an outsider in my world.   *Larch, Water Violet*

☐ Although I have lived so long in the United States
and am well acclimated, I often don't really
feel at home here.   *Water Violet, Scleranthus*

☐ I am afraid of Americans misunderstanding
me because the slight language barrier
makes me unable to share my sense of humor.   *Cerato, Mimulus*

☐ I am angry at the ignorant, racist people
here and have to hold back from becoming
aggressive.   *Holly, Vine, Cherry Plum*

☐ I feel torn between the country where I grew
up and the country that is now my home.   *Scleranthus*

☐ I often think back to my carefree youth in Mumbai.   *Honeysuckle*

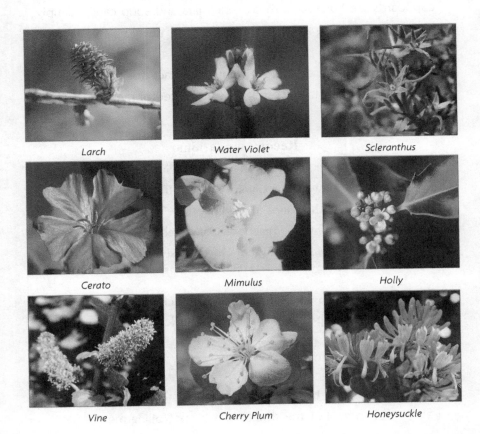

Larch   Water Violet   Scleranthus

Cerato   Mimulus   Holly

Vine   Cherry Plum   Honeysuckle

46. I'm upset that I'm so disorganized.

"The same thing happens each year: I make a resolution to clean things up, get rid of superfluous items, and make a clean break. Then, every time, I get lost in the first few drawers I go through, get absorbed in old letters, and get caught up in memories. And then another day is over without my cluttered apartment looking the least bit different.

"My work room is full of papers, and I waste an incredible amount of time searching when I need specific documents, such as when deadlines need to be met. My attic room is overflowing with a mountain of old newspapers and files that I still want to sort. My kitchen cupboards are bursting with old spice jars and soup cans. I simply can't throw anything away, so I know that I will never be able to clean up everything.

"Now, because the landlord wants the place for himself, I have been given notice. Moving out will be a disaster for me!"

Recommendations

1. Write down your answers to the following question: "Which reactions and Flowers correspond to me?" If too few reactions are found, read the other cases in this chapter.
2. Refer as necessary to the reaction clusters section of this book.
3. Read the additional steps in the "How to Use This Book" chapter.

How do I react, and what Bach Flower patterns are identifiable?

☐ When I think about the move,
I feel paralyzed.   *Star of Bethlehem, Chestnut Bud, Larch*

☐ I feel overwhelmed by my huge amount of stuff.
I am not in control of the situation; it is controlling me.   *Willow*

☐ On the other hand, all these things together form
a sort of nest in which I feel safe.   *Heather*

☐ It is difficult for me to throw away or separate
myself from any of my old things. *Honeysuckle*

☐ I keep making doomed efforts to change the
chaos, but I never get it done. *Chestnut Bud*

☐ I feel like I'm less capable in this regard than most people. *Larch*

☐ I feel as though I'll never manage it. *Gorse, Gentian*

☐ I'm afraid that in my old age I'll completely lose
control of things. *Mimulus*

Star of Bethlehem

Willow

Heather

Honeysuckle

Chestnut Bud

Larch

Gorse

Gentian

Mimulus

47. Help, I can't control my weight!

"I am twenty-three years old and sixty pounds overweight. This is very upsetting to me, but I simply can't get my eating habits under control. When I diet and exercise I do lose weight quickly, but soon I fall back into my old eating habits and gain back the weight.

"As a child, my weight was always normal; my problems began at puberty. I had really bad acne and felt inferior, ugly, and excluded. I suffered terribly from low self-esteem. So to compensate for it, I started stuffing myself with sweets.

"Today I still notice that whenever a problem comes up, I head straight for pastries or chocolate. Since then my weight has gone through this yo-yo pattern. I really have to try to deal with my problems differently, but how?"

Recommendations

1. Write down your answers to the following question: "Which reactions and Flowers correspond to me?" If too few reactions are found, read the other cases in this chapter.
2. Refer as necessary to the reaction clusters section of this book.
3. Read the additional steps in the "How to Use This Book" chapter.

How do I react, and what Bach Flower patterns are identifiable?

☐ I find myself immediately using food as comfort
whenever things get difficult.   *Agrimony, Chestnut Bud*

☐ I am ashamed to be around my thin and fit friends.
I don't even want to do anything with them
anymore.   *Larch, Water Violet*

☐ Then, when I sit alone at home, I get mad at myself
and eat more, simply out of frustration.   *Holly*

☐ Afterward, I realize that I've fallen into the old trap. *Chestnut Bud*

☐ I simply don't have the willpower to say "no,"
even when others encourage me. *Centaury*

☐ I feel completely dependent on food. *Red Chestnut*

☐ If only someone could help me get down to
my desired weight. I can't do it alone! *Willow, Gorse*

Agrimony

Chestnut Bud

Larch

Water Violet

Holly

Centaury

Red Chestnut

Willow

Gorse

48. My horse broke his leg. Do I have to have him put to sleep?

"I grew up around horses. Just like the cowboy in the film *The Horse Whisperer*, I seem to understand horses, and they understand me. So when my mixed-breed horse had his accident—he was a year and a half old, and I'd been intending to break him for riding—it was all the more upsetting. I'd gotten him when he was six months old and bought a share in a pasture so that he could grow up around eight or ten other foals.

"One evening the vet called me and said, 'I have bad news. Your horse is standing on three legs. What should we do?' He diagnosed a complex splintered fracture.

"The chance of healing is minimal. If we tried it, it would be extremely expensive. Breaking him for riding later would be impossible, because the fracture is too complex. It is very rare for an animal to get so badly injured in the pasture. Why did it have to happen to my horse? Everything in me is telling me not to have him put to sleep."

Recommendations

1. Write down your answers to the following question: "Which reactions and Flowers correspond to me?" If too few reactions are found, read the other cases in this chapter.
2. Refer as necessary to the reaction clusters section of this book.
3. Read the additional steps in the "How to Use This Book" chapter.

How do I react, and what Bach Flower patterns are identifiable?

☐ I am stunned, as if struck by lightning.   *Star of Bethlehem*

☐ I am torn between intellect and emotion.   *Scleranthus*

☐ I'm trying not to show how upset I am.   *Cherry Plum, Agrimony*

☐ Every night it breaks my heart when I feel
my horse eating sugar lumps out of my hand
with his velvety mouth.   *Red Chestnut*

☐ I am totally despairing and embittered, because
I know I cannot afford expensive
veterinary care.   *Sweet Chestnut, Willow*

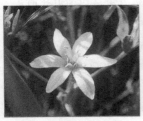
Star of Bethlehem

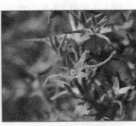
Sclerathus

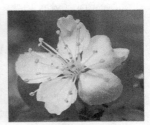
Cherry Plum

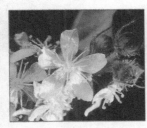
Agrimony

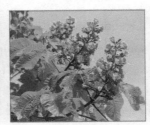
Red Chestnut

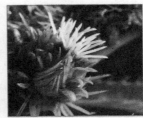
Sweet Chestnut

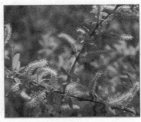
Willow

49. I have to give away my beloved dog. I can't bear it.

"Until now, it wasn't a problem. I just did a bit of house cleaning and I was at home a lot, so I could take good care of Max, the terrier I got seven years ago when he was a puppy.

"But now I've had to take a full-time job because we want to build our own house and we need more money than Hank makes as a crane operator. I was lucky to get a job as a nurse's aide at a hospital in a nearby town.

"But I can't take Max to work with me—I have to give him to my sister-in-law. This breaks my heart! Sure, my sister-in-law has a nice big house with a yard, but she lives a hundred miles away from us. I know Max will be happy there, but it still makes me feel terrible."

Recommendations

1. Write down your answers to the following question: "Which reactions and Flowers correspond to me?" If too few reactions are found, read the other cases in this chapter.
2. Refer as necessary to the reaction clusters section of this book.
3. Read the additional steps in the "How to Use This Book" chapter.

How do I react, and what Bach Flower patterns are identifiable?

☐ I feel guilty, as if I'd thrown out my dog.   *Pine*

☐ I am secretly not sure that the dog will really be
happy with my sister-in-law.   *Gentian*

☐ When I go for a walk, I find myself leaving some
room next to me as if I still had him on the leash.   *Red Chestnut*

☐ Even though I'm no longer a dog owner, I can't bear
to stop subscribing to the dog magazines I used to read.   *Walnut*

☐ Max was like my child—I did everything
for him. No person can replace him for me.
My dog was the only one who loved me
unconditionally.   *Heather, Red Chestnut*

☐ Whenever I see people out walking their dogs,
I get very sad and think of those happy days
I had with my dog.   *Honeysuckle*

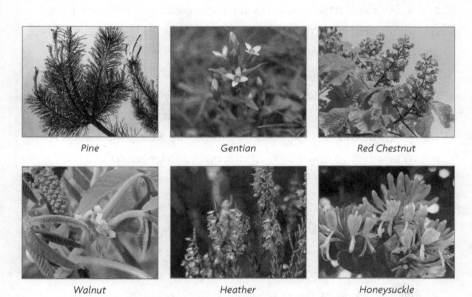

Pine   Gentian   Red Chestnut

Walnut   Heather   Honeysuckle

50. My dog rules this house.

"I was never able to learn what kind of home my Irish setter came from before we got him from the animal shelter. However, it must have been a pretty bad situation, because Bobo is quite traumatized. How do I know this? He's completely uncontrollable.

"On the street he becomes the leader and pulls me in whatever direction he wants to go. If we pass another dog, he strains like mad to break loose and attack. He barks at people passing by and even jumps on them sometimes. Yelling at him doesn't help, and he doesn't obey any commands. The only one in charge is my dog.

"Perhaps I've let him get away with too much, out of compassion for his abused past. I let him sleep on the rug by my bed and give him dog biscuits whenever he begs for them. I just can't deny him anything. I know this isn't the right way to handle a dog. My friends tell me to take him to obedience school, but I don't want to."

Recommendations

1. Write down your answers to the following question: "Which reactions and Flowers correspond to me?" If too few reactions are found, read the other cases in this chapter.
2. Refer as necessary to the reaction clusters section of this book.
3. Read the additional steps in the "How to Use This Book" chapter.

How do I react, and what Bach Flower patterns are identifiable?

☐ I try desperately to control my dog and hold
him back with the leash.   *Vine*

☐ I can't refuse my dog anything. When he begs,
I always give him what he wants.   *Centaury*

☐ I feel like I'm doing something wrong, but I don't
know what to change.   *Cerato*

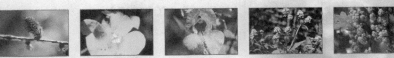

PART 2

The Practical
Application of Bach
Flower Therapy

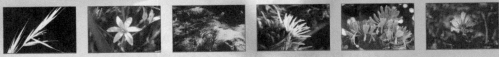

The Reaction Clusters

Elements for Individual
Bach Flower Combinations according
to Mechthild Scheffer

The reaction clusters are combinations of the thirty-eight reactive patterns that can be observed again and again in Bach Flower practice. They facilitate finding the right Bach Flower combinations for your situation.

Naturally, each cluster is one choice among many. In some cases, your personal reaction cluster may not be included here. However, once you have read through the clusters in this book, you probably will be able to identify your own reaction cluster.

SELECTING YOUR PERSONALIZED BACH FLOWER CRISIS COMBINATION

There are four steps in this self-diagnosis system.

Step 1: Describe the actual crisis situation in writing, as concisely as possible, in three or four sentences. In this current situation, how do you most often react?

Step 2: Make your preliminary choices with the help of the questionnaire for the reaction cluster pool. From the twenty-four reactions (cluster pools) in the questionnaire (see page 125), choose two or three that are dominant in the present situation.

Step 3: Specify your choices from the corresponding cluster pool. In each pool you will find between eight and ten reaction clusters (or individual Bach Flower patterns). From among these, choose the ones that best describe your current situation. In this way you will recognize various Bach Flowers that you could use for your crisis combination.

Step 4: Final choice of your Bach Flower crisis combination. The final choice is achieved when you study the diagnosed Flower concepts more deeply, whether by reading or in discussion with an appropriate partner. Flowers that appear multiple times in your chosen clusters definitely should be included in your crisis combination.

Example

Step 1: In a few days, I have to speak with my ex-husband about an allowance for our son's class trip. I know this will be difficult, and I want to steel myself for this discussion.

Step 2: I choose the following clusters from the Reaction Cluster Pool Questionnaire on page 125.

No. 1: "I am fearful."
No. 11: "I react angrily and aggressively."

Step 3: When specifying my choices, I choose from

no. 1: "I am afraid of arguments."   *Mimulus,*
Star of Bethlehem, Agrimony, Centaury

From no. 11 I choose:
"Because I feel as if I've been
treated unfairly."   *Holly, Willow*

Step 4: Since this situation is not new for me, I recognize that all the Flowers I have chosen are still valid. So I take a mixture of all six flowers daily until the day I have to meet with my ex-husband.

DETERMINING WHEN
RESCUE REMEDY IS NEEDED
AS A FIRST STEP

When going through a severe crisis situation, it is often not possible at first to describe one's reactions clearly. If it is difficult for you to determine your cluster pools because you feel at the moment as if everything is applicable, ask yourself whether the following reactions are dominant:

☐ I am in total panic.   *Rock Rose*

☐ I really have to pull myself together.   *Cherry Plum*

☐ I feel as if I've been run over by a train.   *Star of Bethlehem*

☐ I must do something immediately.   *Impatiens*

☐ I feel dizzy.   *Clematis*

This is the rescue cluster. If three or more of these reactions are present in you at the moment, take only Rescue Remedy in a glass of water for several days before you return to the reaction cluster questionnaire.

REACTION CLUSTER POOL QUESTIONNAIRE

What are the main features of my reaction?

Please choose only the two or three statements that are most applicable to your *current* situation.

- ☐ 1. I am fearful.
- ☐ 2. I feel stressed.
- ☐ 3. I am overly sensitive and too easily hurt.
- ☐ 4. I am uncertain and have doubts.
- ☐ 5. It is difficult for me to make decisions.
- ☐ 6. I react inconsistently.
- ☐ 7. It is difficult for me to concentrate.
- ☐ 8. I am too flexible—it's difficult for me to say no.
- ☐ 9. I am drained and exhausted.
- ☐ 10. I feel hurt and injured.
- ☐ 11. I react angrily and aggressively.
- ☐ 12. I react by being controlling, stubborn, or intolerant.
- ☐ 13. I put myself under time pressure.
- ☐ 14. I overdo things and don't know when to stop.
- ☐ 15. I have feelings of worthlessness.
- ☐ 16. I am withdrawing into myself.
- ☐ 17. I cannot react—I am numb.
- ☐ 18. I am despondent—I give up.
- ☐ 19. I have no motivation, and I feel depressed and sad.
- ☐ 20. I feel subservient.
- ☐ 21. I reproach myself.
- ☐ 22. I cannot let go.
- ☐ 23. I am harsh and rigid with myself.
- ☐ 24. I feel overwhelmed and powerless.

1. I am fearful.

☐ I fall into a panic and lose perspective.   *Rock Rose*

☐ I am afraid of . . . (please insert concrete situations,
for example, illness, dental surgery, public speaking)   *Mimulus*

☐ I have groundless fears that I can't understand.   *Aspen*

☐ I'm afraid of losing self-control and doing things
I don't want to do.   *Cherry Plum*

☐ I'm afraid of losing control of my
own thoughts.   *Cherry Plum, White Chestnut*

☐ I'm worried about a relative/friend/pet or
someone else.   *Red Chestnut*

☐ I'm afraid of the unknown future.   *Aspen, Mimulus*

☐ I'm fearful of being afraid.   *Cherry Plum, Aspen*

☐ I'm afraid of dirt, diseases, germs, and so on.   *Aspen, Crab Apple*

☐ I'm afraid of "bad vibes."   *Aspen, Crab Apple*

☐ I'm afraid of disappointment.   *Mimulus, Gentian, Star of Bethlehem*

☐ I'm afraid of being psychically injured.   *Mimulus, Holly*

☐ I'm afraid to show my true feelings.   *Mimulus, Agrimony*

☐ I'm afraid of people seeing through me.   *Mimulus, Pine, Agrimony*

☐ I'm afraid of making mistakes.   *Mimulus, Pine, Cerato, Larch*

☐ I'm afraid of failure.   *Mimulus, Larch, Willow*

☐ I fear confrontations.   *Mimulus, Star of Bethlehem,
Agrimony, Centaury*

☐ I'm afraid of my own unconscious feelings.   *Cherry Plum, Agrimony*

☐ I'm afraid of being alone.   *Mimulus, Heather*

☐ I'm afraid of hurting others unintentionally.   *Mimulus, Holly, Pine*

☐ I'm afraid of making the wrong decision.   *Mimulus, Cerato, Scleranthus*

☐ I'm afraid of giving up or
changing relationships.   *Mimulus, Chicory, Honeysuckle, Walnut*

☐ I'm afraid of exhaustion and strain.   *Mimulus, Olive, Hornbeam*

☐ I'm afraid of close, intimate contact.   *Mimulus, Water Violet*

☐ I'm afraid of falling short
and missing out.   *Mimulus, Heather, Chicory, Holly*

☐ I have a fear of flying.   *Rock Rose, Cherry Plum, Willow, Honeysuckle*

☐ I am superstitious.   *Aspen*

2. I feel stressed . . .

☐ When I don't have all the details in order.   *Rock Rose, Crab Apple*

☐ When I panic and lose my perspective.   *Rock Rose*

☐ When I have to deal with something new.   *Rock Rose, Mimulus*

☐ When I hear bad news or have to watch
people quarreling.   *Rock Rose, Agrimony, Aspen*

☐ When I have to hold myself back
too much.   *Rock Rose, Cherry Plum, Rock Water*

☐ When I have taken on too many responsibilities.   *Rock Rose, Elm*

☐ When I am becoming too impatient.   *Impatiens, Chestnut Bud*

☐ When I get burned-out.   *Rock Rose, Olive*

☐ Because I am inwardly insecure.   *Rock Rose, Scleranthus, Cerato*

☐ Because my expectations of myself
are too high.   *Rock Rose, Rock Water, Vervain, Elm*

☐ Because I don't pick up on things
quickly enough.   *Rock Rose, Rock Water, Chestnut Bud*

☐ Because too much is required of me.   *Elm, Willow, Vine*

☐ Because I can't keep a promise.   *Rock Rose, Oak*

3. I am overly sensitive and too easily hurt.

☐ I expect things of other people, and I get
disappointed when they don't follow through.　　*Chicory, Heather*

☐ I have an allergic kind of reaction to
disorganization in small details.　　*Crab Apple, Rock Rose*

☐ I have a difficult time taking criticism.　　*Larch, Beech*

☐ Loud noises, bright lights, strong smells, and so forth
quickly become too much for me.　　*Mimulus*

☐ I very quickly become irritated, upset, and angry.　　*Holly, Rock Rose*

☐ Conflicts in my surroundings are very
stressful for me.　　*Agrimony, Mimulus*

☐ Antagonism throws me offtrack.　　*Vine, Larch*

☐ I am very sensitive to the weather.　　*Scleranthus*

☐ I pick up moods strongly from my surroundings
and get exhausted quickly.　　*Aspen*

☐ I'm afraid of someone opposing me; I would
rather give in right away.　　*Centaury, Mimulus*

☐ I am so sensitive that I need to be
handled with kid gloves.　　*Star of Bethlehem, Heather*

☐ When my plans are criticized, I become insecure.　　*Walnut, Beech*

☐ I empathize too strongly with others—
it's difficult to distance myself.　　*Red Chestnut, Walnut*

4. I am uncertain and have doubts . . .

☐ When others are observing me.   *Centaury, Larch, Mimulus*

☐ Because I want to make everything
   right for everyone.   *Cerato, Centaury, Agrimony*

☐ Because I don't know exactly what I want.   *Cerato, Wild Oat*

☐ Because I don't trust myself enough.   *Cerato, Larch, Mimulus*

☐ Because I consult and discuss things with
   other people too much.   *Cerato, Walnut*

☐ Because I doubt that I can handle
   increased responsibility.   *Elm, Gentian, Mimulus*

☐ Because I don't trust my own decisions.   *Scleranthus, Larch*

☐ Because I have done a lot of things
   wrong in the past.   *Pine, Cerato, Honeysuckle*

☐ Because I always let other people
   make me question myself.   *Chestnut Bud, Cerato, Walnut*

☐ Because I don't know whether
   my decision is the right one.   *Gentian, Scleranthus, Wild Oat*

☐ I will use any means possible to
   hide my insecurity.   *Agrimony, Vervain, Cherry Plum*

☐ I doubt whether I am good enough.   *Larch, Pine, Gentian*

☐ I doubt whether I have the strength to
   complete my task.   *Hornbeam, Elm*

☐ I doubt that everything will go well.   *Gentian, Aspen*

5. It is difficult for me to make decisions . . .

☐ Because I don't want to make a commitment.   *Wild Oat*

☐ Because I always waver back and forth
between two possibilities.   *Scleranthus*

☐ Because I don't trust my decision-making abilities
and don't want to make another mistake.   *Cerato, Chestnut Bud*

☐ Because I am afraid of not being able to face
the consequences of my decisions.   *Scleranthus, Mimulus, Elm*

☐ Because I am preoccupied by an old,
unresolved problem.   *Honeysuckle, Walnut*

☐ Because I am inwardly dependent on another
person and cannot make any free decisions. *Red Chestnut, Walnut*

☐ Because I would rather leave decisions up to
stronger and smarter people.   *Larch, Centaury*

☐ Because I think fate will make the
decision for me.   *Centaury, Willow, Aspen*

☐ Because a great deal depends on the
decision.   *Scleranthus, Mimulus, Rock Rose*

☐ Because I am afraid that I won't be
able to reverse the decision
once it is made.   *Scleranthus, Wild Oat, Mimulus*

☐ Because I'm overwhelmed by the
great number of choices.   *Scleranthus, Wild Oat, Willow*

6. I react inconsistently . . .

☐ Because I respond to all influences, like a leaf
blown around in the wind.   *Scleranthus*

☐ Because I don't trust my own opinions.   *Cerato*

☐ Because I always believe a better possibility is
waiting for me.   *Wild Oat*

☐ Because I let small things distract me.   *Crab Apple*

☐ Because I want to pursue several different
ideas at the same time.   *Wild Oat, Scleranthus*

☐ Because my thoughts are unfocused.   *Clematis*

☐ Because vague fears and worries
always hold me back.   *Aspen, Mimulus*

☐ Because internally I am not fully
committed to the matter.   *Cerato, Wild Oat, Walnut*

☐ Because I want to do everything right.   *Agrimony, Scleranthus,*
                                                              Centaury

☐ Because I always question my own decisions.   *Cerato, Scleranthus*

☐ Because I can't see a clear goal yet.   *Wild Oat*

7. It is difficult for me to concentrate . . .

☐ Because I am mentally worn out
and unmotivated. *Olive, Hornbeam*

☐ Because I have too many things going on
in my mind. *Hornbeam, White Chestnut*

☐ Because I lose interest or let myself
get distracted too easily. *Scleranthus, Wild Oat, Chestnut Bud*

☐ Because I'm not sure what I really want. *Cerato, Wild Oat*

☐ Because I get mentally exhausted very easily. *Olive, Hornbeam,
Cerato, Chestnut Bud*

☐ Because I am hyperactive in my thoughts. *White Chestnut*

☐ Because I lose myself in the details. *Crab Apple*

☐ Because I want to take on too many things
at once. *Wild Oat, Impatiens*

☐ Because my inner reactions are hectic
and too driven. *Impatiens, Vervain*

☐ Because I space out easily. *Clematis*

☐ Because I quickly get nervous
and then lose my perspective. *Rock Rose*

☐ Because I am always thinking about something else
in the back of my mind. *Clematis, White Chestnut, Wild Oat*

8. I am too flexible—it is difficult for me to say no . . .

☐ Because I don't want to hurt anyone.   *Centaury, Agrimony, Pine*

☐ Because I don't have a definite goal.   *Centaury, Wild Oat*

☐ Because I want to be tolerant.   *Beech, Centaury*

☐ Because I'm afraid of confrontation.   *Mimulus, Centaury, Agrimony*

☐ Because I don't know what I should actually do.   *Cerato, Walnut*

☐ Because I feel guilty when I say what I really want.   *Pine, Vine*

☐ Because I can't deal well with
strong personalities.   *Centaury, Aspen, Larch*

☐ Because I don't have the strength for it.   *Centaury, Olive*

☐ Because I trust others more than I trust myself,
and I let them tell me what to do too often.   *Larch, Cerato*

☐ I must learn to assert myself more.   *Vine, Centaury*

☐ I feel guilty once I've gotten my way.   *Vine, Pine*

9. I am drained and exhausted . . .

☐ Because suddenly everything has happened at once. *Elm*

☐ Because for a long time I've had to bear far too much. *Olive, Oak*

☐ Because the everyday rat race drains
and cripples me. *Olive, Hornbeam*

☐ Because the pressure to expand my mind
keeps increasing, and I am always pushing at my
mental boundaries. *Olive, Cerato, Chestnut Bud, Hornbeam*

☐ Because it takes a great deal of energy
for me to hide my anxiety. *Olive, Larch, Mimulus*

☐ Because I have taken on too many responsibilities
and find it difficult to delegate. *Olive, Elm*

☐ Because a lot of what I have to do is a strain. *Olive, Vervain*

☐ Because I have such high expectations of myself,
and I don't give myself any breaks. *Olive, Rock Water, Vervain*

☐ Because I'm good-natured and have taken on
too many extra tasks. *Olive, Centaury*

☐ Because I don't have any more motivation. *Gentian, Wild Rose*

☐ Because I'm depressed and don't believe
I will be successful anymore. *Olive, Mustard, Gentian*

10. I feel hurt and injured . . .

☐ Because I am being wronged. *Holly, Vervain*

☐ Because even when I'm detached, I still feel
pulled in different directions. *Walnut, Scleranthus, Red Chestnut*

☐ Because I have been betrayed. *Holly, Willow*

☐ Because I believe others should be
more appreciative. *Holly, Chicory*

☐ Because I feel unjustly criticized. *Beech, Willow*

☐ Because I feel as if I've done everything wrong. *Cerato, Walnut, Pine*

☐ Because I haven't yet recovered from
an unexpected confrontation. *Star of Bethlehem, Holly, Agrimony*

☐ I mustn't show how hurt I am. *Holly, Agrimony, Cherry Plum*

☐ I'm hurt because I meant well but I was
misunderstood. *Willow, Chicory*

☐ Because something didn't go as I expected,
I feel sorry for myself and want to
withdraw from the situation. *Chicory, Water Violet*

☐ Thoughts of revenge are spinning around in my mind,
and this makes me feel guilty. *Holly, White Chestnut, Pine*

☐ I am painfully lovesick. *Sweet Chestnut, Star of Bethlehem, Holly, Willow*

☐ I feel rejected and undervalued. *Holly, Larch*

☐ I am offended and react by feeling hurt. *Holly, Chicory*

11. I react angrily and aggressively . . .

☐ Because I absolutely want to get my own way.   *Holly, Vine*

☐ Because I am impatient.   *Holly, Impatiens*

☐ Because I feel as if I've been treated unfairly.   *Holly, Willow*

☐ Because I don't show my feelings for a
long time, and then I suddenly explode.   *Holly, Cherry Plum*

☐ Because I think I am being deceived.   *Holly, Aspen*

☐ Because something doesn't work as I'd
imagined it would.   *Chicory, Holly*

☐ Because I feel helpless and overwhelmed.   *Heather, Holly, Elm*

☐ Because I feel abandoned and powerless.   *Holly, Willow*

☐ Because in the past I was abused and exploited.   *Honeysuckle,*
Holly, Willow

☐ Because people don't understand me,
and no one believes me.   *Holly, Willow, Cerato*

☐ Because I'm afraid of being hurt and want to
protect myself.   *Mimulus, Holly*

☐ Because I think my partner has done
something wrong.   *Beech, Holly*

☐ Because I have put up with too much
for too long.   *Centaury, Holly, Vine*

☐ Because I've made a mistake and can't admit it.   *Pine, Holly*

12. I react by being controlling, stubborn, or intolerant . . .

☐ Because I believe I have to force others to
   act in their own interest.   *Vervain, Vine*

☐ Because I want to assert my own ideas
   at any cost.   *Vine, Holly, Vervain*

☐ Because I want to convert others to my way of thinking.   *Vervain*

☐ I try to get my ideas implemented by indirect
   methods or through other people.   *Vine, Chicory*

☐ Because I always want to get my way, I am
   accused of being egotistical.   *Vine*

☐ In order to reach my goals, I cleverly manipulate
   other people.   *Vine, Chicory*

☐ I have trouble with people in authority.   *Vine*

☐ I hold others to a high standard of
   order and integrity.   *Crab Apple, Beech*

☐ I criticize others when they don't adhere
   to my values.   *Beech, Rock Water*

☐ I react angrily when others do not keep up
   with my pace.   *Holly, Impatiens*

☐ I become obstinate about an issue and won't
   give it up, on principle.   *Vine, Rock Water*

☐ On principle, I stick to any decision that
   has been made.   *Oak, Rock Water*

☐ I put myself and others under pressure
   because I am so sure of my own ideas.   *Rock Water, Vervain*

13. I put myself under time pressure . . .

☐ Because I want to get everything done
immediately.   *Impatiens, Vine*

☐ Because I want to put everything behind
me as quickly as possible.   *Impatiens, Aspen, Water Violet*

☐ Because I have burdened myself with
too many tasks.   *Elm, Rock Water, Vervain*

☐ Because I'm good-natured and take
on too many tasks for others.   *Centaury, Chestnut Bud*

☐ Because my enthusiasm for something
makes me lose perspective.   *Impatiens, Vervain*

☐ Because I have too many things going
on in my head at once.   *Impatiens, Wild Oat,*
White Chestnut, Crab Apple

☐ Because I have to meet deadlines.   *Impatiens, Vine, Willow*

☐ Because I'm afraid time is slipping
through my fingers.   *Impatiens, Willow, Aspen*

☐ I berate myself when I don't get
my work done.   *Impatiens, Larch, Pine*

14. I overdo things and don't know when to stop . . .

☐ Out of enthusiasm for some idea. *Vervain*

☐ In my thoughts and feelings. *Sweet Chestnut*

☐ In eating, drinking, shopping, and so on. *Vervain, Heather*

☐ In using my strength. *Vervain, Olive*

☐ When I am in love. *Holly, Vervain, Sweet Chestnut*

☐ Because of my overactive sense of duty. *Oak, Pine, Vervain*

☐ Because I am very ambitious. *Vine, Sweet Chestnut*

☐ Out of empathy. *Red Chestnut, Vervain*

☐ Out of perfectionism. *Vervain, Rock Water*

☐ I am addicted to doing things for
the sake of doing them. *Impatiens, Vervain*

☐ At work (workaholic). *Chicory, Vervain*

☐ In my concern for others. *Vervain, Red Chestnut*

15. I have feelings of worthlessness . . .

☐ Because I feel hopelessly inferior.   *Larch, Gorse, Willow*

☐ Because I don't feel capable of following
through on a commitment.   *Larch, Walnut, Cerato*

☐ Because I always let myself be persuaded
too easily.   *Larch, Centaury*

☐ Because my mind doesn't pick up
on things very quickly.   *Larch, Chestnut Bud, Hornbeam*

☐ Because of my appearance.   *Beech, Larch, Crab Apple*

☐ Because I'm afraid that others are more
capable than I am.   *Larch, Mimulus*

☐ Because I'm afraid of no longer being able
to fulfill my responsibilities.   *Elm, Mimulus*

☐ Setbacks erode my self-esteem.   *Larch, Gentian*

☐ I don't let my feelings of
inferiority show.   *Agrimony, Larch, Cherry Plum*

☐ When I feel inferior, I react by being
defiant or petulant.   *Larch, Vine*

16. I am withdrawing into myself . . .

☐ Because I feel inwardly distant from others.   *Water Violet*

☐ Because I have less self-confidence than others,
   I hide in the background.   *Water Violet, Larch*

☐ Because I am very sensitive.   *Water Violet, Star of Bethlehem*

☐ Because I'm very critical of other people.   *Water Violet, Beech*

☐ Because I do everything more quickly than other
   people and can't work in a team.   *Impatiens*

☐ Because I'm not very good at making conversation,
   I'm critical of myself.   *Water Violet, Pine, Larch*

☐ Because I don't believe anything will change,
   I continually withdraw.   *Water Violet, Gorse, Gentian*

☐ Because I'm shy, I talk as little as possible.   *Mimulus, Water Violet*

☐ Because I am afraid of making a fool
   of myself.   *Mimulus, Larch, Beech*

☐ Because I'm not as quick-witted
   as others.   *Mimulus, Star of Bethlehem, Larch*

☐ Because I am so preoccupied with myself
   and my own world.   *Heather, Clematis*

☐ Because talking with other people
   is very draining.   *Aspen, Red Chestnut, Olive*

☐ Because my thoughts are currently
   preoccupied by something else.   *Clematis, White Chestnut*

☐ Because I'm disappointed, sad, and embittered.   *Gentian, Willow*

☐ Because I cannot approach other people impartially,
people think I'm arrogant. *Water Violet*

☐ Because small things about other people disturb me
greatly, for example, their way of speaking,
clothing, or body scent. *Beech, Crab Apple, Water Violet*

☐ Because I'm afraid of taking on
new responsibilities. *Mimulus, Elm, Water Violet*

☐ Because I am seldom able or willing
to be spontaneous. *Chicory, Cherry Plum, Agrimony*

☐ Because I'm afraid of letting others
latch on to me. *Water Violet, Mimulus, Star of Bethlehem*

☐ Because I don't want to be bothered
with other people's problems. *Chicory, Heather, Water Violet*

☐ Because I am afraid of confrontations. *Water Violet,
Agrimony, Mimulus*

☐ Because as a child I had to witness many conflicts.
Star of Bethlehem, Agrimony, Willow

☐ People think I am indecisive
and capricious. *Water Violet, Scleranthus, Wild Oat*

☐ Others accuse me of not letting them get a word in
edgewise and pull away from me. *Heather, Water Violet, Willow*

17. I cannot react. I am numb . . .

☐ Because I expect too much of myself.   *Rock Water, Vervain*

☐ Because I haven't gotten over a
   traumatic experience.   *Star of Bethlehem*

☐ Because I've had bad experiences.   *Star of Bethlehem,*
Gentian, Honeysuckle

☐ Because I can't stop thinking about
   a particular issue.   *White Chestnut, Chestnut Bud*

☐ Because I am afraid of being exploited.   *Honeysuckle, Vine, Chicory*

☐ Because I am so thin-skinned that I take in
   everything, and it paralyzes me.   *Aspen, Scleranthus,*
Star of Bethlehem

☐ Because I don't know what to do anymore.   *Sweet Chestnut,*
Wild Oat, Cerato

☐ Because when I try to implement
   my ideas, I always run up against
   the same obstacles.   *Vervain, Gentian, Chestnut Bud*

☐ I am deeply depressed, but I don't know why.   *Mustard*

18. I'm despondent—I give up . . .

☐ Because I can't handle any more strokes
of bad luck.   *Honeysuckle, Willow, Star of Bethlehem*

☐ Because I believe it's my fate. What I hoped for
is "not meant to be."   *Gentian, Aspen, Willow*

☐ Because I have lost all hope of change.   *Gorse*

☐ Because life no longer gives me any joy.   *Gorse, Wild Rose, Willow*

☐ Because deep down, I still don't know
what I really want.   *Gentian, Wild Oat*

☐ Because deep down I don't believe I deserve
anything better.   *Pine, Gentian*

☐ Because obstacles keep being thrown in my way,
over and over.   *Gentian, Willow, Chestnut Bud*

☐ Because I am completely burned out.   *Olive, Gorse*

☐ When the first difficulty arises, I immediately become
pessimistic.   *Gentian*

☐ I am at a psychological low point.   *Mustard, Gentian*

19. I have no motivation, and I feel depressed and sad . . .

☐ Because my difficult past still haunts me. *Honeysuckle, Willow, Mustard*

☐ Because after many bad experiences, I no longer believe there is any good in humanity. *Wild Rose, Gorse, Gentian*

☐ Because I haven't yet recovered from a disappointment. *Star of Bethlehem, Gentian, Willow*

☐ Because I don't have any perspective. *Gentian, Gorse*

☐ I'm exhausted and apathetic. *Olive, Wild Rose, Mustard*

☐ I'm sad and self-critical. *Mustard, Pine*

☐ I am mourning the loss of a beloved friend, relative, partner, or pet. *Mustard, Red Chestnut, Honeysuckle*

☐ In my sadness, I retreat further and further into my own world. *Mustard, Water Violet, Clematis*

☐ I feel powerless and distraught. *Willow, Sweet Chestnut*

☐ I am pessimistic and embittered. *Gentian, Willow*

☐ My sadness follows me even into my dreams. *White Chestnut, Mustard, Gentian*

☐ Because I'm very worried about someone else. *Red Chestnut, Gentian*

☐ Because I've lost something that was precious to me. *Willow, Honeysuckle*

20. I feel subservient . . .

☐ Because I am too good-natured and always give
   people things.   *Centaury, Pine*

☐ Because I am too deeply involved in all my relationships.   *Chicory*

☐ To the moods and whims of other people.   *Walnut, Willow,*
                                            Star of Bethlehem

☐ To the mood and atmosphere
   of my surroundings.   *Agrimony, Aspen*

☐ To a former partner.   *Honeysuckle, Red Chestnut*

☐ Because I don't know how to make decisions by myself.   *Cerato*

☐ Because I can't influence the situation.   *Willow*

☐ Because I feel stifled.   *Willow, Vine*

☐ Because I believe I have to be a victim.   *Willow, Pine*

☐ To what other people want.   *Centaury, Agrimony*

☐ To a person to whom I am very
   closely connected.   *Red Chestnut, Walnut*

21. I reproach myself . . .

☐ Because I am so critical.   *Pine, Beech*

☐ For not having any opinion of my own.   *Pine, Cerato*

☐ For not living up to my responsibilities.   *Pine, Elm*

☐ For having made an unavoidable mistake.   *Pine, Beech*

☐ For not being able to say no.   *Pine, Centaury*

☐ For having missed a once-in-a-lifetime
   opportunity.   *Pine, Honeysuckle*

☐ For being egotistical and thinking too much of
   myself.   *Pine, Heather*

☐ I am so ashamed, I'd just like to crawl
   into a hole.   *Pine, Water Violet*

☐ It depresses me to think about how someone
   must be feeling.   *Pine, Red Chestnut*

☐ I regret being so mean.   *Pine, Vine, Agrimony*

22. I cannot let go.

☐ I have to get over the shock before I let go.   *Star of Bethlehem*

☐ I'm afraid to dive into something new.   *Rock Rose, Mimulus*

☐ I'm afraid of starting over.   *Mimulus, Aspen, Walnut*

☐ I'm afraid of hurting other people by letting go.   *Agrimony, Pine*

☐ I still haven't worked through things
    that happened in the past.   *Honeysuckle, Beech, Willow*

☐ I want everything to stay the way it always
    used to be.   *Honeysuckle, Chicory*

☐ I feel as if I'm tied to another person
    with an invisible umbilical cord.   *Red Chestnut, Walnut*

☐ I'm worried about losing face.   *Mimulus, Agrimony*

☐ I don't know whether the decision to separate
    is the right one.   *Cerato, Scleranthus*

☐ I don't know how things will go after
    the separation.   *Wild Oat, Aspen*

23. I'm harsh and rigid with myself.

☐ I am too harsh and strict with myself. I expect
   too much self-discipline.   *Rock Water*

☐ When I let myself indulge in something,
   I feel guilty.   *Rock Water, Pine*

☐ I force myself to keep going at any price;
   it's almost masochistic.   *Rock Water, Vine, Oak*

☐ I try to keep my feelings under rigid control.   *Cherry Plum,*
                                                           Rock Water

☐ I want to be perfect, so I criticize myself
   mercilessly.   *Rock Water, Beech*

☐ My everyday life goes back and forth between
   self-discipline and chaos.   *Rock Water, Clematis*

☐ I always want to be strong, so I demand too much
   of myself and then get exhausted.   *Rock Water, Olive, Oak*

☐ When I can't live up to my own high standards of
   discipline, I feel ashamed.   *Oak, Pine*

24. I feel overwhelmed and powerless . . .

☐ Because I still haven't recovered from
a trauma. *Star of Bethlehem, Willow*

☐ Because unfair things happen to me. *Willow, Vervain*

☐ Because I have to do things that I don't
actually want to do. *Willow, Vine, Cerato*

☐ Because I can't show my feelings
in my position or role. *Willow, Agrimony, Cherry Plum*

☐ Because something has been taken away from me. *Vine, Willow*

☐ Because I don't have the same opportunities
as others. *Honeysuckle, Willow*

☐ Because I feel weaker and smaller
than other people. *Willow, Larch*

☐ Because I have less strength as I get older. *Hornbeam,*
Honeysuckle, Olive, Gorse

How to Prepare
Bach Flower Combinations

THE BACH FLOWER REMEDIES

The thirty-eight Bach Flower Concentrates are concentrated flower tinctures. They are free from side effects and are compatible with all other forms of therapy, in both mainstream and alternative medicine. The majority of the original Bach Flowers are still collected in the wild at locations favored by Edward Bach.

Bach Flower Remedies are sold in full-strength bottles called stock bottles; they are diluted before they are taken.

DOSAGE AND APPLICATION

You can take your Bach Flower combination in two different ways.

The Water Glass Method

For distinct, acute conditions and for quick daily treatment, take two drops of each chosen Bach Flower Remedy (or four drops of Rescue Remedy) in a glass of water and drink it in small sips throughout the day.

The Mixing Bottle Method

For long-term treatment, add three drops of each chosen Bach Flower Remedy (six drops of Rescue Remedy) to a 30-mL dropper bottle. Fill the bottle with distilled water. To better preserve it, fill the bottle with three-fourths water and one-fourth 90-proof spirits (cognac, brandy, or the like).

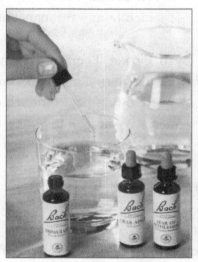 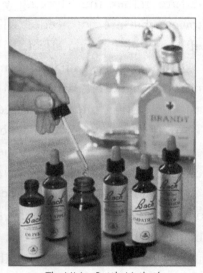

The Water Glass Method   *The Mixing Bottle Method*

The Standard Dose

The standard dose is four drops from the bottle, four times daily, for about three weeks. You can vary the frequency of dosage and number of drops without any risk. There is no danger of overdosing.

NUMBER OF FLOWERS, AND HOW TO COMBINE THEM

In general, six different types of Flowers are used in combination, but in an acute crisis it sometimes seems impossible to limit the selection in this way. In such cases, as many as ten Flowers can be used.

If, in the heat of a crisis, you are in no condition to determine your best options, it may be better to take only Rescue Remedy in water for a few days and then reconsider the composition of your personal Flower combination. When in doubt, consulting with someone experienced in Bach Flower Therapy can be very helpful.

If you cannot decide between two Flowers, add both to the mixture rather than forcing yourself to decide between them. Flowers that are not needed will not generate any resonance and will therefore have no effect.

In the progress of long-term Bach Flower Therapy, the most important patterns emerge with increasing clarity, and it becomes easier to restrict oneself to three to five Flowers per combination. This reduced number of Flowers makes it simpler to grasp the concepts of the Flowers and the spiritual misunderstandings that lie behind them.

Any Flower can be combined with any other Flower. Initially, some Flower concepts might seem incompatible (for example, "being unable to say no" while at the same time "wanting to get one's way at any price"). But the problem is often precisely that apparently opposite conditions are internally experienced simultaneously, thus creating inner tension. If both Flowers are added to the mixture, the two conditions can come back to equilibrium and one's overall condition can be harmonized.

BASIC PRINCIPLES OF FLOWER SELECTION

The only thing that counts is what is acute at this moment. Choose only those Flowers that correspond exactly to the negative psychic condition you are experiencing *now*.

If a given psychic condition fits well with your personality but you are not experiencing it *right now*, this Flower does not belong in your crisis combination.

Spontaneous choices may be highly informative, because they provide momentary views into your unconscious psychic landscape; but only by considering the psychic concept lying behind these choices should you determine whether a spontaneously chosen Flower should actually be added to your remedy.

Physical conditions should *not* be taken into account in the selection of Bach Flowers.

DURATION OF THERAPY

Every Bach Flower should be taken for as long as it is effective—that is, until the corresponding condition has been harmonized. You will be able to feel when this harmony has been achieved because your need to keep taking this combination will perceptibly diminish.

In acute crises, in which your psychic condition may change quickly, the effect may be experienced within the space of hours or a few days. The water glass method is best suited for adapting the composition of your Flower combination to these quickly changing needs.

Once you have established your key behavior patterns, prepare your combination in a dropper bottle. This will be enough for eighteen to twenty-eight days. When you have emptied the first bottle, consider whether the composition of the combination corresponds to your then current psychic condition and change a few Flowers if necessary. The total number of dropper bottles you will need depends on the complexity of your personal development process. Therapy may last from two to eighteen months.

INITIAL REACTIONS

If multiple dreams emerge during the initial period of taking Bach Flower Remedies, or if old feelings and symptoms that are perceived as negative become stronger, it is an indication that the process of change is under way. Observe these reactions as part of the purification process.

If you find the initial reaction very stressful, you can reduce your dosage, if necessary, to just a drop a day. Taking Rescue Remedy in addition has also been proven effective. To keep the process in motion, we recommend from experience that you do not completely stop the therapy.

The empowering statements have been proven to be especially effective for getting through the initial reactions.

THE EMPOWERING STATEMENTS

The empowering statements strengthen the positive potential of the Bach Flowers. They express the harmonic condition that you wish to reach by taking your remedy. Say these short sentences to yourself while taking your Bach Flower mixture. Repeat them from memory or write them on a piece of paper that you can tape to your mirror or somewhere around your work area.

How to Determine Your Personal Empowering Statement

To put together your own empowering statement, write all the statements that correspond to the Flowers chosen for your remedy (see the individual Flower pages in the final chapter of the book).

For example, if your Flower mixture is Olive, Vervain, Larch, and Honeysuckle, the following are the sentences you can choose from:

Olive

I am at rest.
I am strengthened.
I recover.

Vervain

   I let it go.

   I give space to others.

   I pace my energy.

Larch

   I can do it.

   I want to do it.

   I do it.

Honeysuckle

   I live today.

   I look to the future.

   I take the next step.

Now, using these sentences in whatever order you like, put together your personal empowering statement. **Your empowering statement will always consist of three sentences,** but you do not need to choose a sentence from each Flower. The only important thing is that the formula should feel good for you now. The wording of the sentences should not be changed.

Your personal empowering statement may be:

Vervain	I let it go.
Honeysuckle	I look to the future.
Olive	I recover.

After a few days, you may feel the need to put together a new empowering statement.

The 38 Individual Bach Flower Remedies, Plus Rescue Remedy

This chapter presents each of the thirty-eight individual Bach Flower Remedies in more detail. The table that begins on the facing page provides an overview of the entire Bach Flower system, indicating the focus and function of each individual Flower, plus Rescue Remedy. The pages that follow explore the spiritual misunderstanding mediated by each Bach Flower, list the positive behaviors and emotional states that each Flower promotes, and offer three empowering statements for use with each Flower.

The Way from Misunderstanding to Change

- Behind each negative Bach Flower reaction pattern there exists, unconsciously and fundamentally, a positive impulse—a constructive goal.
- Through spiritual misunderstandings, people become separated from their Inner Guidance and cannot reach this constructive goal. (Often, instead, they arrive at its opposite.)
- By gaining insight into the misunderstanding, one can restore the connection to one's Inner Guidance.
- Through this, one becomes able to change behavior and reach the original, unconsciously desired goal.

AN OVERVIEW OF THE BACH FLOWER SYSTEM

BACH FLOWER	KEY WORDS	REHARMONIZATION PROCESS
1. Agrimony	The Honesty Flower	From pretend harmony to inner peace
2. Aspen	The Psychic Flower	From dark premonitions to conscious sensitivity
3. Beech	The Tolerance Flower	From know-it-all to better understanding
4. Centaury	The Service Flower	From passive service to active service
5. Cerato	The Intuition Flower	From indecisiveness to inner certainty
6. Cherry Plum	The Openness Flower	From overload to relaxation
7. Chestnut Bud	The Learning Flower	From superficiality to experience
8. Chicory	The Relationship Flower	From demanding love to giving love freely
9. Clematis	The Reality Flower	From escaping reality to living in reality
10. Crab Apple	The Cleansing Flower	From compulsive order to inner order
11. Elm	The Responsibility Flower	From self-worth crisis to inner confidence
12. Gentian	The Belief Flower	From doubt to trust
13. Gorse	The Hope Flower	From giving up to going forth

BACH FLOWER	KEY WORDS	REHARMONIZATION PROCESS
14. Heather	The Identity Flower	From needy child to understanding adult
15. Holly	The Heart-Opening Flower	From hard-heartedness to generosity
16. Honeysuckle	The Past Flower	From the past to the present
17. Hornbeam	The Vitality Flower	From listlessness to mental freshness
18. Impatiens	The Time Flower	From impatience to patience
19. Larch	The Self-confidence Flower	From self-restriction to self-unfolding
20. Mimulus	The Courage Flower	From fear of the world to trust in the world
21. Mustard	The Light Flower	From soul pain to soul grandeur
22. Oak	The Endurance Flower	From unflagging duty to inner commitment
23. Olive	The Regeneration Flower	From exhaustion to inner renewal
24. Pine	The Self-acceptance Flower	From self-reproach to self-respect
25. Red Chestnut	The Cutting-free Flower	From symbiosis to autonomy
26. Rock Rose	The Liberation Flower	From panic to heroic courage
27. Rock Water	The Flexibility Flower	From dogmatic discipline to going with the flow

BACH FLOWER	KEY WORDS	REHARMONIZATION PROCESS
28. Scleranthus	The Balance Flower	From inner conflict to inner equilibrium
29. Star of Bethlehem	The Comfort Flower	From shock to reorientation
30. Sweet Chestnut	The Salvation Flower	Through darkness to light
31. Vervain	The Enthusiasm Flower	From fanatic to light bearer
32. Vine	The Authority Flower	From controlling to cooperation
33. Walnut	The Manifestation Flower	From vacillation to inner steadfastness
34. Water Violet	The Communication Flower	From isolation to interaction
35. White Chestnut	The Thought Flower	From mental merry-go-round to stillness
36. Wild Oat	The Vocational Calling Flower	From seeking to finding
37. Wild Rose	The Zest for Life Flower	From apathy to devotion
38. Willow	The Destiny Flower	From resenting fate to taking personal responsibility
39. Rescue Remedy	The Emergency Remedy	From shock and trauma to calm reassurance

1. Agrimony
The Honesty Flower

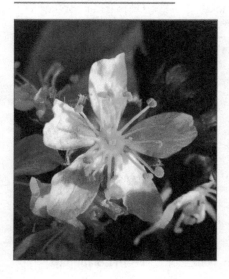

Promotes:

❧ Honorable behavior toward self and others

❧ Understanding of your own needs and requirements

❧ Readiness to confront conflicts

THEME:
READINESS TO CONFRONT CONFLICTS

Key Symptoms

Attempts are made to conceal disturbing thoughts and an inner restlessness behind a cheerful face and nonchalance.

Recognize the spiritual misunderstanding...

In striving for harmony and an ideal world, you unconsciously ignore the fact that you live in a world of dualities. In this world, the two poles—beautiful and ugly, struggle and repose, and so on—are both part of the equilibrium.

In order not to have to perceive the dissonant, less-appealing aspects of your life and of yourself, you often filter them out of your mind, either suppressing them or finding distractions from them. An artificial, beautiful harmony is constructed, and you try by all possible means to preserve it. However in doing this, you lose connection with your own personality and your Inner Guidance.

Since you do not know your true Self, you also have no true contact with your fellow humans, and thus never experience true empathy.

. . . And correct it.

It is important to see that all rose-colored glasses and all false-harmony constructs must sooner or later shatter on the rocks of reality.

When you are ready to deal with all the aspects of life, you will recover contact with your Inner Guidance. You will then gain the power to live a more authentic life. This will bring joy, and you will experience moments of true harmony more and more frequently.

∽

Empowering statements:

    ❧ I feel peaceful.

    ❧ I am honest.

    ❧ I reveal my true Self.

2. Aspen

The Psychic Flower

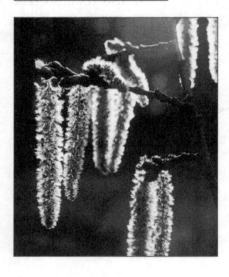

Promotes:

- ℣ Ability to distinguish between different levels of consciousness

- ℣ Constructive use of one's talent for perception

THEME: THIN SKIN

Key Symptoms

There are inexplicable, vague worries, apprehensions, or secret fears of impending danger.

Recognize the spiritual misunderstanding . . .

You are open to the world and have highly developed perceptions. Unconsciously, you want to use them. Unfortunately, your emotional antennae are extended so far outward that you have lost contact with your Inner Guidance.

The boundaries of your personality are becoming too permeable. You often unconsciously take in others' thoughts and feelings from the surrounding energy field and are unable to process them intellectually. This generates free-floating anxiety, manifesting in fearful fantasies. It becomes increasingly difficult to decide what is real and what you have created in your mind.

. . . And correct it.

To recover the connection to your Inner Guidance, you must learn to increase awareness of your personal boundaries.

Practice distinguishing whether feelings or thoughts are really your own, or if you are unconsciously absorbing them from those around you. Put your intellect to work, and with its help determine what is realistic and what is unrealistic.

Then you can use your finely tuned perceptions constructively for your own development and also to help other people.

Empowering statements:

✿ I am protected.
✿ I am centered.
✿ I am strong.

3. Beech
The Tolerance Flower

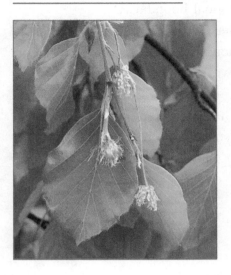

Promotes:

℞ Empathy and tolerance toward yourself, other people, and situations

THEME:
TOLERANCE AND CRITICISM

Key Symptoms

There is a tendency to be overcritical and intolerant and to lack empathy and sensitivity toward others and toward yourself.

Recognize the spiritual misunderstanding . . .

You have an unconscious desire to make the world perfect. Erroneously, you attempt this using your own personal criteria as the standard, thus closing yourself off from other people.

At these times, you are separated from your Inner Guidance and from perspective of the Greater Whole, which makes it impossible to have a real connection with other people. Therefore, encouraging other people to improve themselves yields no results, and they reject you.

... And correct it.

When you reopen your heart to the Greater Whole and start respecting situations as they are, you will regain connection to your Inner Guidance. That will enable you to observe situations with more empathy and judge things more objectively.

You will find the right way to approach arguments. Suddenly, constructive discussions will start taking place, and possibilities for positive development in the face of problems will become apparent.

Empowering statements:

- ❧ I accept.
- ❧ I'll meet you halfway.
- ❧ I see the possibilities.

4. Centaury
The Service Flower

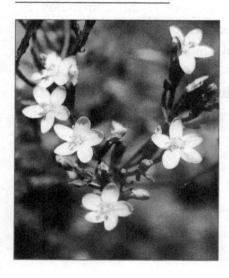

Promotes:

℠ Strengthening of the Self

℠ The ability to set limits

℠ Recognition and formulation of your own needs

THEME:
BEING UNABLE TO SAY NO

Key Symptoms

One cannot say "no"; there is a weakness of will and hypersensitivity to the wishes of others.

Recognize the spiritual misunderstanding . . .

You have a strong feeling for the community of all beings, and unconsciously you want to make a personal contribution to the Greater Whole—like a small child who is overjoyed at being allowed to help older siblings in a demanding common task.

But at the same time, your awareness of your own personality and Inner Guidance, and your ideas of what you want and do not want, are not strongly developed. Therefore you react without reflection, almost automatically, to the wishes of stronger personalities. In doing this, you do not consider whether it is helpful to your own Life Plan or to the Greater Whole. You never say no, and your natural need to serve others is often exploited.

... And correct it.

It is important for you to understand that the most important service that you have to perform is the unfolding of your own Life Plan. Through this, you automatically serve the development of the Greater Whole! In order to do this, it is important to develop your own personality and, above all, your force of will. With the help of your Inner Guidance, you can then decide in each case whether your help supports a mutual process of growth or whether you would merely be encouraging inappropriate behavior in others.

You will gain respect when you are able to refuse requests, and the tasks you do undertake will be all the more valued.

෨෨

Empowering statements:

෨ I stand up straight.
෨ I am who I am.
෨ I do what I want.

5. Cerato
The Intuition Flower

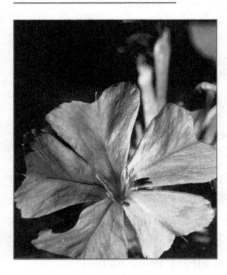

Promotes:

- S Development of your own opinion

- S Confidence in making decisions

- S Trust in your own intuition

THEME:
TRUST IN YOUR OWN OPINION

Key Symptoms

There is a feeling of insecurity and too little confidence in one's own opinions and intuition.

Recognize the spiritual misunderstanding . . .

You want to have a deeper understanding of things and to do everything well and "right." In attempting this, you assume—in many cases, because of what you've been taught—that this is not a simple task. Therefore, you don't trust your Inner Guidance when it suddenly presents you with ideas and solutions, and you ignore them.

Instead, you turn outward and ask other people what you should do. You hold the erroneous belief that they know better than you, and often you end up doing things that don't fit into your own Life Plan. Therefore, you have disappointing experiences, you are ridiculed, and you become increasingly unsure of your own ideas.

. . . And correct it.

It is important to recognize that you must take full responsibility for your own Life Plan. This can happen only when you turn inward and nurture contact with your Inner Guidance.

If you practice trusting your first impressions and going by them, you will learn to use your intuitive gifts successfully—for yourself and for others.

Empowering statements:

- ✄ I trust myself.
- ✄ I pay attention to my first impressions.
- ✄ I make my own decisions.

6. Cherry Plum

The Openness Flower

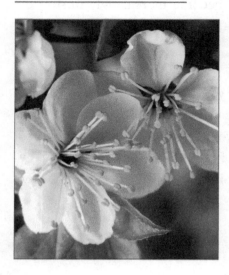

Promotes:

≈ The ability to express feelings at the right time and to the right degree

≈ A more relaxed interaction with your own world of feelings

THEME:
EMOTIONAL PRESSURE

Key Symptoms

It is difficult to relax internally; there is a fear of losing control over your own emotions and of acting irrationally.

Recognize the spiritual misunderstanding . . .

You have the unconscious desire to "strong-arm" your life. You may have learned early in life that spontaneously expressing your emotions puts you at a disadvantage. For this reason, you believe that you have to control your emotions.

When the pressure from your emotions is too great, you boil over. By doing so, you cause yourself to be disliked and thus become increasingly fearful of your own emotions.

... And correct it.

It is important to understand that emotions are inevitable. They are the tools that your Inner Guidance uses to push you further along on your life path.

Confront your fear and reconnect with your inner world of feelings. Stating clearly how you really feel will open contact with your own Inner Guidance and with the hearts of other people.

Share your feelings. It will enrich everyone involved.

Empowering statements:

- ❧ I am courageous.
- ❧ I open myself.
- ❧ I let flow what wants to flow.

7. Chestnut Bud

The Learning Flower

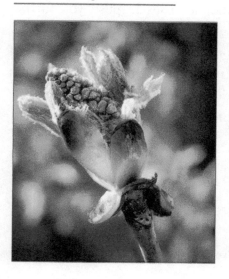

Promotes:

∞ Attentiveness and
observation

∞ Recognition of undesired
automatic reaction patterns

∞ Constructive learning from
experience

THEME: REPEATED MISTAKES

Key Symptoms

There is a tendency to repeat the same mistakes over and over, because experiences are not really digested and not enough is learned from them.

Recognize the spiritual misunderstanding . . .

You have the unconscious desire to learn as much and as fast as possible. Consequently, you ignore the fact that a step taken easily and effortlessly on the mental level will require complete immersion and detailed concentration when applied in the practical domain. Only successful physical manifestation of an idea can make an action into a good experience that you can draw upon later.

Since your thoughts are always jumping ahead, you don't pay enough attention to the details of practical application. You react automatically and by habit and you cannot hear the impulses of your Inner Guidance. You always come up against the same barrier but do not know why.

... And correct it.

To reach a goal, you must dedicate 100 percent of your attention to all the things that you do, for as long as it takes, until the process is totally completed. In these moments, you are connected to your Inner Guidance.

Consequently, when a mistake has happened, you can retrace exactly when and why it took place, and you'll know what to change in the future.

Thus you learn new things continually, and your life's development will be greatly accelerated.

Empowering statements:

∞ I am paying attention.
∞ I listen carefully.
∞ I am learning.

8. Chicory
The Relationship Flower

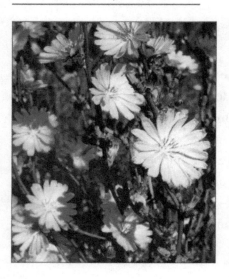

Promotes:

⁞ Readiness to accept your own psychic needs and to fulfill them yourself, directly

THEME:
INTERFERENCE AND MANIPULATION

Key Symptoms

Feeling a lack of love and appreciation, you develop a manipulative attitude, which leads you to interfere consciously or unconsciously in the lives of others.

Recognize the spiritual misunderstanding . . .

You have an unconscious desire to love selflessly and to be loved, but it's probable that you have never in your life experienced true, unconditional love. Therefore, you have tried to "sell" yourself with accomplishments (good grades, being dutiful, and so on). Thus you have lost contact with your Inner Guidance and your true ability to love has been blocked.

This behavior pattern continues today. You try to ensure the loving devotion of others with your achievements. In doing this—

often with the best of intentions—you become involved in the Life Plans of other people.

When others do not respond as you had hoped, you are disappointed.

. . . And correct it.

It is important to recognize that just like every other person, you are allowed to have your own psychic desires fulfilled without having to pay for them on some level. By doing so, you will regain connection to your Inner Guidance. You will be able to accept the fact that every person must live his or her own life.

You stop interfering and learn to trust that love is given when you act and love selflessly according to your Inner Guidance.

Empowering statements:

    ❖ I give freely.
    ❖ I am nourished by my source.
    ❖ I am loved.

9. Clematis
The Reality Flower

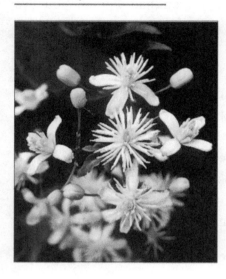

Promotes:

- Acceptance of your life's reality

- Presence

- The realization of ideas

THEME:
RELATIONSHIP TO REALITY

Key Symptoms

You are mentally absent, daydream, and have no real interest in what is going on in your immediate surroundings.

Recognize the spiritual misunderstanding . . .

With your strong power of imagination, you unconsciously try to find and cocreate paradise on Earth with others. When the conditions of real life are in strong contrast with this paradise, you immediately drift away, fleeing to realms of fantasy and ideas.

In these moments, you draw away from the reality of life and thus also from your Life Plan and your Inner Guidance. You invest your energy on the wrong levels, which leaves insufficient energy for accomplishing concrete tasks in the present.

... And correct it.

It is important to understand that an idea is only a constructive contribution to the Greater Whole if it fits sensibly within our material reality and can be realized.

Reflect upon your ideas and put what is sensible into action, step-by-step. By doing so you will reconnect with your Inner Guidance, and your creativity can unfold constructively. You will gain more inner power, and more and more facets of your Life Plan can manifest easily.

Empowering statements:

- ❧ I am awake.
- ❧ I see clearly.
- ❧ I create.

10. Crab Apple
The Cleansing Flower

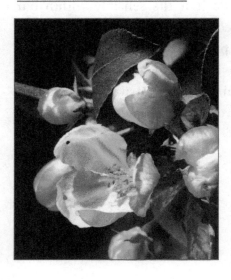

Promotes:

♛ Connection to your physical nature

♛ Acceptance of your body

♛ Seeing and setting priorities

THEME:
ORDER AND PURITY

Key Symptoms

There is a feeling of being unclean, impure, or infected, inside and out. You have an obsession with details and order.

Recognize the spiritual misunderstanding . . .

Your unconscious wish is to bring more purity and order to the world, but you do not realize that on the earthly plane there can never be perfect, enduring order and purity. Life is a process of constant creation and destruction.

Because you are so preoccupied with maintaining your vision of perfection, external order, and purity, your connection with Inner Guidance gets lost. You become too fixated on details, and lose sight of greater connections and priorities in your Life Plan.

. . . And correct it.

It is important to turn your attention from the microcosm to the macrocosm—and to understand that you are a part of the Greater Whole.

You should understand that nature continually goes through processes of ordering and purification, and these processes also take place in individual people, on a small scale. All you need to do is allow them to unfold.

Thanks to this new perspective, you are automatically reconnected with your Inner Guidance. You will regain your sense of proportion and priorities. You will be able to make progress with your personal purification and reordering in a more loving and natural manner.

Empowering statements:

    ✇ I feel good.
    ✇ I accept myself as I am.
    ✇ I see what's really important.

11. Elm

The Responsibility Flower

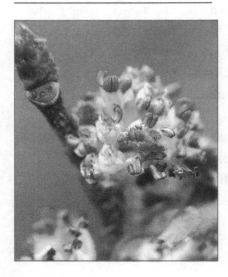

Promotes:

℅ Awareness of your own need for healing and the limits of your abilities

℅ A realistic approach to your responsibilities

THEME: OVEREXTENDING

Key Symptoms

There is, temporarily, an overwhelming sense of not being equal to one's tasks or responsibilities.

Recognize the spiritual misunderstanding . . .

Since, in your role in life, you want to be equal to all your responsibilities, you believe that you should be able to manage by yourself, expecting superhuman things of yourself. In doing this, you are ignoring impulses from your Inner Guidance that are telling you to rest. You stretch the boundaries of your individual abilities, and when a moment of weakness comes, despite your better instincts, you are convinced that you are fundamentally unequal to your responsibilities.

. . . And correct it.

In actual fact letting your own Life Plan unfold—with all of its human facets—is the most important responsibility you have. You do not need to demand anything superhuman of yourself. Your Inner Guidance will tell you exactly when your personal limits should be respected.

When you listen to this voice, you will be able to modify your tasks in such a way that you will be sure of being adequate—while still meeting your own personal needs.

Empowering statements:

- ∞ I do what I can.
- ∞ I receive help.
- ∞ I can manage.

12. Gentian
The Belief Flower

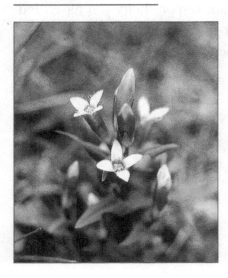

Promotes:

   ◈ Optimism

   ◈ Trust in the positive forces in human life

   ◈ A constructive attitude toward life

THEME:
DISCOURAGEMENT AND SKEPTICISM

Key Symptoms

Your tendency is to be skeptical, doubting, pessimistic, and easily discouraged.

Recognize the spiritual misunderstanding . . .

Unconsciously, you want to believe and trust like a child. But in life's ups and downs, when things turn out to be different from what you expected, you become discouraged and in disappointment, you draw back from your Inner Guidance.

To protect yourself from further disappointment, you become skeptical or have negative expectations and thus constantly block contact with your Inner Guidance. Sometimes it is even inwardly satisfying when your negative predictions turn out to be correct. Your life becomes increasingly devoid of joy.

... And correct it.

What is important now is to change your fundamental perspective in a positive, constructive, creative direction. This will restore connection to your Inner Guidance.

Please understand, every natural development takes place in waves. Every apparent setback or standstill actually serves to stabilize what has been attained so far and provides helpful orientation for the next exciting step in development.

Empowering statements:

- ❧ I am confident.
- ❧ I expect the positive.
- ❧ I know everything works out right.

13. Gorse
The Hope Flower

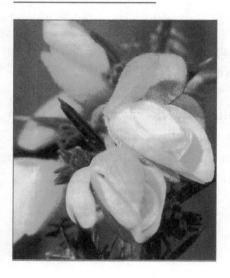

Promotes:

& Hope and creativity in long-term, difficult life situations

THEME: RESIGNATION

Key Symptoms

Hopelessness, resignation, and an "Oh, what's the use?" attitude.

Recognize the spiritual misunderstanding . . .

Your unconscious desire is for continual growth and a joyful unfolding of life. But long-lasting, difficult life conditions, for example unemployment or chronic illness, have restricted your perspective on life so much that you see possibilities disappearing and believe you can't go any further. You are resigned.

As a consequence, you erroneously set up passive resistance to your Inner Guidance. Therefore, you can no longer recognize the new constructive possibilities or the opportunities for spiritual development inherent in every situation. Your flow of life energy dwindles.

. . . And correct it.

The fact is that as long as there is life, there is hope.

Try to find out what new insights or other facets of your Life Plan might be developed as a result of the current situation. Approach these ideas creatively and begin bringing one or two of them into reality. This will bring joy, and the life flow will start up again.

Empowering statements:

☙ I stand tall.
☙ I am filled with hope.
☙ I see new opportunities.

14. Heather

The Identity Flower

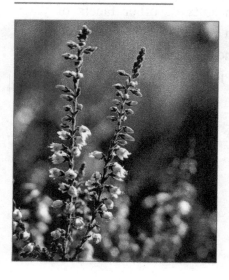

Promotes:

- Ծ Mature handling of your own needs

- Ծ Ability to empathize with and understand others

- Ծ Readiness to enter into relationships

THEME: NEEDINESS

Key Symptoms

Self-centeredness, preoccupation with your own troubles and affairs, a constant need for attention: "the needy child."

Recognize the spiritual misunderstanding . . .

When a baby receives inadequate care and attention, her sense of identity may not develop sufficiently. She unconsciously wants to compensate for this deficiency, to be taken care of, and somehow to fill the resulting psychic void.

People with this psychic condition erroneously turn only outward for help. In doing this, they do not establish contact with their Inner Guidance and do not recognize what they truly need.

Under these conditions, a sense of the needs of others cannot be developed. You may talk nonstop and be unaware of what your partner in conversation is really saying. Thus, true exchange cannot take place. Sooner or later, this will irritate and push away any conversation partner, resulting in the exact opposite of what you desire.

... And correct it.

To regain connection to your Inner Guidance, it is important to learn to stop living in your world as its lonely center and begin living as part of a great network of people in lively exchange, in a constant give-and-take.

Only through this exchange can you get to know who you actually are and receive what you really need. And so your identity will unfold.

Empowering statements:

- ❧ I feel safe.
- ❧ I receive all that I need.
- ❧ I am growing.

15. Holly
The Heart-Opening Flower

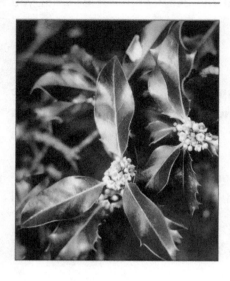

Promotes:

⊠ Generosity of spirit

⊠ Bigheartedness

⊠ Understanding of human nature

THEME:
EMOTIONAL VULNERABILITY

Key Symptoms

On the emotional level, you are irritable, distrusting, and easily hurt or offended. Jealousy, envy, or hate may develop.

Recognize the spiritual misunderstanding . . .

You pursue a high emotional ideal, unconsciously seeking Divine Love. But since people with these selfless and strong feelings are often misunderstood, hurt, or disappointed early in life by the all-too-human world, you have come to believe that something is wrong with your emotions.

You close off your heart, guard against the impingements of your Inner Guidance, and react with irritation, mistrust, or hosility when other people express their feelings. Your positive feelings swiftly turn into the opposite, becoming anger, spite, vindictive-ness, or jealousy. You hurt other people with these emotions, but more than anything else, you hurt yourself.

... And correct it.

It is helpful to become aware of the difference between fundamen-tal feelings (for example, love for a partner) and transient emo-tional reactions (for example, anger at someone who forgets to return a phone call). These transient reactions can vary in intensity depending on their type, but they do not change your fundamental feelings.

Open your heart to your Inner Guidance! With its help, you will be much better able to evaluate the feelings and reactions of others, and will be able to react on the right level in each case. In the free space thus created, you can finally fully express your own strong feelings and find an appropriate response. You will love and be loved.

Empowering statements:

> ✂ I am full of joy.
> ✂ I am connected.
> ✂ I am loving.

16. Honeysuckle

The Past Flower

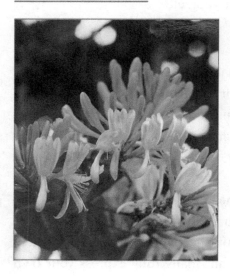

Promotes:

   ❖ Realistic and constructive processing of past events

   ❖ Orientation in the present

THEME:
OVERCOMING THE PAST

Key Symptoms

Consciously or unconsciously, you refuse to work through certain events in the past.

Recognize the spiritual misunderstanding . . .

You have an unconscious wish to preserve and protect the positive values of life. Consequently, you misguidedly try to hang on to only the good experiences of the past, editing out any undesirable experiences. These good experiences from the past become your standard for judging events in the present.

In these moments, you are cut off from your Inner Guidance and you live less and less in the here and now. The unfolding of your Life Plan stagnates.

. . . And correct it.

It is important to become clear that the river of life always keeps flowing. Every new event has a unique experiential quality that cannot be compared absolutely, side by side, with past events.

When you are ready to consider all your experiences—good and bad—and to go into every new situation without holding back, then you will regain connection with your Inner Guidance. With its help, every experience can be adequately processed. You can take along the essence of experience that has been distilled by you on your life's path, and also pass it on to other people.

Empowering statements:

❀ I live today.
❀ I look to the future.
❀ I take the next step.

17. Hornbeam

The Vitality Flower

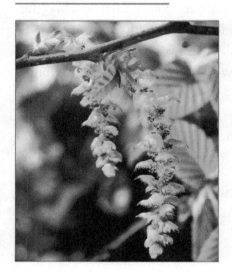

Promotes:

- ⚮ A sense of rhythm and variety

- ⚮ The mental readiness to give up rote activities that no longer serve you and to react more spontaneously with your inner impulses

THEME: MENTAL ATROPHY

Key Symptoms

The "Monday-morning" feeling; no energy for daily obligations, but somehow things get done.

Recognize the spiritual misunderstanding . . .

You want to, or must, perform tasks, and this requirement has usurped your spontaneity and enjoyment of life. Your daily routine has too much rigid structure, which reduces the possibility of receiving inspiration from your Inner Guidance.

Because you always know exactly what is going to happen next, your curiosity and motivation are lost. You keep needing more and more energy to pull yourself together and get ready for your daily tasks. Often—almost ritually—you seek external stimulants such as tea, coffee, or cigarettes to help you get moving. Since this stimulation is not lasting, your feeling of fatigue increases.

. . . And correct it.

It is important to recognize and accept that the stream of life does not proceed in a uniform line. Each hour has its own energetic qualities suited to a specific form of activity that ought to come naturally.

The conscious perception of these varying rhythms and energetic qualities will help you to grant yourself greater spontaneity and creativity in your everyday life. Then inspiration from your Inner Guidance will return. You will be motivated once again—perhaps you will even look forward to an exciting workday when you wake up each morning.

Empowering statements:

- ❧ I feel fresh.
- ❧ I have energy.
- ❧ I enjoy working.

18. Impatiens

The Time Flower

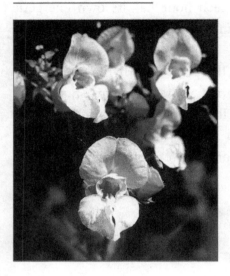

Promotes:

- ɪ Patience with oneself

- ɪ Understanding of different human reaction patterns

THEME: IMPATIENCE

Key Symptoms

Impatience and irritability; you react very quickly.

Recognize the spiritual misunderstanding . . .

In your unconscious effort to continue your life's development, you restrict yourself to a one-sided, purely quantitative view of time. Sticking to a misguided idea that you must arrive at your goal as quickly as possible, you look to neither right nor left. Instead, you strive to squeeze as much as you can into the shortest time possible.

This distances you from your Inner Guidance. Therefore, you cannot relate to the inner rhythms of your fellow human beings, which may be slower than your own; you fail to perceive life's larger time cycles, and you lose your sense of time quality. You end up racing past other people and racing through your life.

... And correct it.

If you become aware that all people progress together in a great flow of time, you will reconnect with your Inner Guidance and regain contact with your fellow humans. This will help you develop a feeling of the right moment to use favorable circumstances—efficiently but effortlessly—to reach your goals.

Empowering statements:

- ⊗ I have time.
- ⊗ I am patient.
- ⊗ I am relaxed.

19. Larch
The Self-confidence Flower

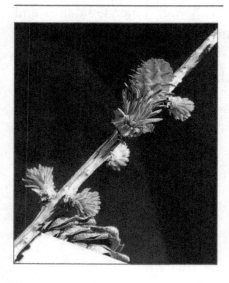

Promotes:

℣ Recognition and realistic evaluation of one's own strengths and weaknesses

℣ Self-reliance

℣ Courage for self-realization

THEME:
SELF-ESTEEM AND SELF-RELIANCE

Key Symptoms

Feelings of inferiority; lack of self-confidence leads one to expect failure.

Recognize the spiritual misunderstanding . . .

You have the unconscious wish to do everything as well as possible.

As a child, you often were confronted with prejudice (for example, "Girls can't do that!"), or else your achievements were compared to those of other people (siblings, parents, archetypes) to teach you various lessons. Therefore, logically, you could only ever do worse than other people. Contact with your Inner Guidance has atrophied. You have not been able to form any appropriate standards of achievement that correspond to your own natural abilities and your Life Plan.

As an adult, you continue to set external standards for yourself. You feel wronged, a failure, and you underestimate yourself. Your outlook on life is correspondingly subdued.

. . . And correct it.

It is important now to let go of all external standards. By doing this, you will restore contact with your Inner Guidance.

Your individual Life Plan will only set tasks for you that you are, in principle, able to fulfill. But you must summon the confidence to go your own way and to trust that you can do it. Only then will your success be lasting.

Empowering statements:

⍟ I can do it.
⍟ I want to do it.
⍟ I do it.

20. Mimulus
The Courage Flower

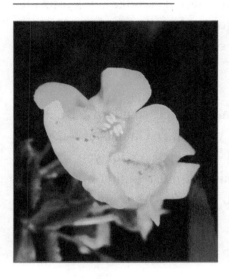

Promotes:

& Personal bravery

& Courage to take things in hand

& Calmer handling of your own sensitivity

THEME: FEAR

Key Symptoms

You have specific, well-defined fears; you are shy and timid and have many small anxieties.

Recognize the spiritual misunderstanding . . .

Unconsciously, you want someone to hold your hand as you go through life, like a child with its mother. But because you have lost the connection to your Inner Guidance, you feel as if that hand isn't there. "Oh, the world is so big . . . and I am so small!"

From this perspective, obstacles seem larger and events seem more significant than they really are. You become unnecessarily frightened, overreact, and shy away from important developmental steps in life.

... And correct it.

What is important now is to remember that you have Inner Guidance. Hand in hand with this guidance, you can practice going through the anxiety-provoking situations. In doing so, you will make the surprising discovery that you can actually master any life situation—entirely in your own way.

Step-by-step you will gain inner strength and become master of your own fate. You will then be able to follow your own path through the world, without fear.

Empowering statements:

❧ I am brave.
❧ I dare.
❧ I step forward.

21. Mustard

The Light Flower

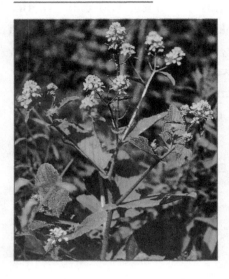

Promotes:

- & The ability to understand the interplay between collective emotions and your own emotions

- & Psychic maturity and cheerful calmness

THEME:
DEJECTION FOR NO REASON

Key Symptoms

Deep sadness; periods of melancholy that suddenly appear and vanish for no apparent reason.

Recognize the spiritual misunderstanding . . .

Your unconscious wish to live as part of the Greater Whole makes you very open to the world and to impersonal, collective emotional currents.

When collective sadness—caused, for example, by war or natural disasters—falls into resonance with your own unconscious reservoir of sadness, you are enveloped by these strong collective feelings as if by a huge black cloud. Contact with your Inner Guidance and your surrounding world is incapacitated. You suffer along passively until the collective emotional weather has cleared.

. . . And correct it.

You cannot prevent the occurrence of such conditions by yourself, but you can allow these dark times to be fruitful for your own Life Plan. The first step to take is to observe the context of your ups and downs more attentively. If you trust in your Inner Guidance and resolve to go through dark periods completely consciously, then you will not be swept up so helplessly but instead will continue participating in life.

By these means you will become more mature and will experience all feelings more deeply—including life's happy moments.

Empowering statements:

> ❧ I feel uplifted.
> ❧ I am happy.
> ❧ I am in the light.

22. Oak

The Endurance Flower

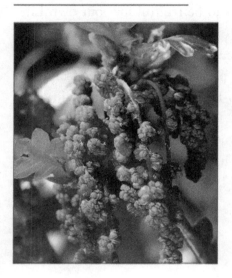

Promotes:

⚭ The ability to let go

⚭ Enjoyment and ease when doing work

⚭ A sense of your own needs and limitations

THEME:
STICKING TO IT, NO MATTER WHAT

Key Symptoms

The exhausted soldier who fights on bravely, never giving up.

Recognize the spiritual misunderstanding . . .

Unconsciously wanting to keep your word no matter what happens, you mistakenly feel obligated, at any price, to stand by decisions you have made. For example, you feel that you must keep a promise you have made, even if conditions have changed so much in the meantime that it now makes no sense to do exactly what you said you would do.

In doing this, you are ignoring the promptings of your Inner Guidance. As if you had sworn an internal oath of allegiance, you hold duty-bound to your word, despite changing conditions, and thus sap yourself of energy. Your work achievements imperceptibly decline, and the situation becomes dissatisfying for everyone involved.

... And correct it.

Please realize that the most important duty you have is the unfolding of your own individual Life Plan.

To reach this goal, sometimes you will inevitably have to reconsider previously made decisions—with the help of your Inner Guidance—and respond to changing conditions. Thanks to this, your decisions will remain realistic and you will be able to reach the goals you have set for yourself more calmly, without constant stress.

Empowering statements:

    ❧ I relax.
    ❧ I manage things easily.
    ❧ I feel free.

23. Olive

The Regeneration Flower

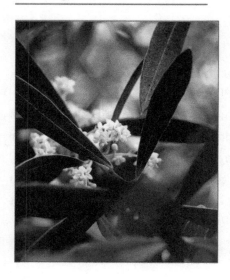

Promotes:

⁎ Awareness of how to use your energy reserves and resources economically

⁎ The rebuilding of energy reserves from past, exhausting experiences

THEME:
DENIAL OF EXHAUSTION

Key Symptoms

Complete exhaustion; physical and mental fatigue; "it's all too much."

Recognize the spiritual misunderstanding . . .

Unconsciously, you want to do everything that you do completely, all the way. Consequently, you erroneously assume, like a child, that you have inexhaustible personal energy reserves. Children have not yet developed the awareness that one's total spiritual, emotional, and physical energy are not all 100 percent available at every moment.

Since you are ignoring the wisdom of your Inner Guidance, you give out your energy in double handfuls. Again and again you end up totally exhausted, with your energy account overdrawn. The unfolding of life cannot continue.

... And correct it.

It is important for you to learn, with the help of your Inner Guidance, how to use your energy reserves economically. Your bodily intuition will make you aware of how to regulate your energy at any given moment: when you have to conserve energy, and when you need time to regenerate.

Once you have learned to use your energy in the correct amounts, you will be able to continue along your life's path without running up against exhaustion.

Empowering statements:

⚮ I am at rest.

⚮ I am strengthened.

⚮ I recover.

24. Pine

The Self-acceptance Flower

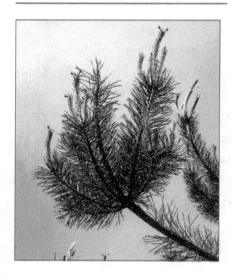

Promotes:

❦ Self-acceptance

❦ Proper processing of inappropriate guilt feelings and
self-accusations

THEME: GUILT FEELINGS

Key Symptoms

Self-reproach and inappropriate guilt feelings.

Recognize the spiritual misunderstanding . . .

Just like everyone else, you want to feel inwardly accepted and
to feel that you belong somewhere. But for a long time—maybe
even since birth—you have had the feeling that you are "not right,"
or are in some way guilty. Erroneously, you believe that you are
unwelcome and not entitled to help from a Higher Power or from
your own Inner Guidance.

Instead, you live with the unconscious feeling of having to earn
your right to existence by performing self-sacrificing tasks. You
may feel so guilt laden that you accept unjustified accusations of
guilt without any reflection, or even unconsciously attract them.

... And correct it.

Now is the time to make the decision to rethink things completely. Call upon your Inner Guidance. Realize that you are not an intruder into this life. Like every human being, you have an automatic right to existence. Simply by virtue of having been born, you have a part in the Greater Whole.

Understand that with your Life Plan you are fulfilling a unique role in which no one else can take your place. Feel how liberating this realization is.

Empowering statements:

❧ I am allowed to do it.
❧ I am forgiven.
❧ I am freed.

25. Red Chestnut

The Cutting-free Flower

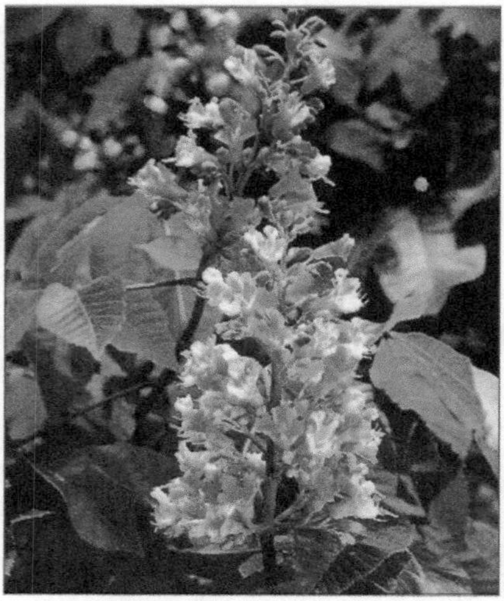

Promotes:

- Release from emotional snares and dependency
- Building the boundaries of one's own personality

THEME:
EMPATHY AND BOUNDARIES

Key Symptoms

You are more concerned about the well-being of other people than about your own well-being; you are too emotionally connected to another person.

Recognize the spiritual misunderstanding . . .

At the root of this problem, there is the unconscious human yearning to merge with the Greater Whole.

On the human plane, this can be imagined as follows: As a baby, you felt at ease only when your mother felt at ease. Therefore, you unconsciously bound yourself to her feelings, sensing and experiencing them as if they were your own.

This pattern—unconsciously preserved—often leads later to a lack of clear boundaries between yourself and someone else's personality. Therefore, you also lack a clear perception of your own Inner Guidance and Life Plan. You cannot distinguish whose feelings you are actually feeling. You do not only absorb unconscious feelings of anxiety from other people, you also project your own feelings onto others. Consequently, you do not feel really free and independent internally.

... And correct it.

Your task is to decisively build your connection with your Inner Guidance and develop greater self-awareness.

Practice intentionally distancing yourself from external emotions and experiencing your own emotions very consciously. By doing this, you will find the right balance between independence and empathy.

⚡

Empowering statements:

⚡ I am myself.
⚡ I stay with myself.
⚡ I am me and you are you.

26. Rock Rose
The Liberation Flower

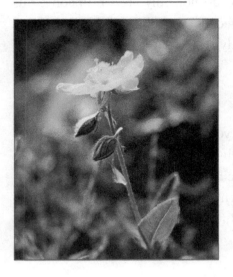

Promotes:

& Spiritual presence

& Constructive handling of stressful demands

THEME: INTERNAL PANIC

Key Symptoms

Reactions are panicky and you have overwhelming feelings of terror.

Recognize the spiritual misunderstanding...

A child who cries and cries until he forgets what he is crying about ends up completely disoriented. The same happens to you when you are flooded by overly intense feelings of anxiety. Your Inner Guidance seems disconnected. You no longer know which end is up—you are overwhelmed by anxiety and can't even sense yourself anymore.

However (and perhaps you know this already), in such intense states of energetic excitement, your Inner Guidance is much closer to you than usual.

... And correct it.

At some point, you must decide not to let your energies keep spinning around in panic but to concentrate your full attention upon yourself and open yourself without reservation to your Inner Guidance. This interrupts the panic. Sometimes you will even go beyond your capabilities and suddenly find you can mobilize super-human powers.

Rock Rose makes it possible for you to make a quick decision to call upon your Inner Guidance. For this reason, it is an integral ingredient in Rescue Remedy.

Empowering statements:

    ❧ I will survive.
    ❧ I know things will go well.
    ❧ I see things clearly.

27. Rock Water

The Flexibility Flower

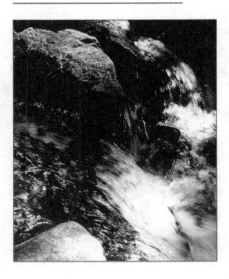

Promotes:

⟠ The ability to let go internally

⟠ Spiritual openness and flexibility

⟠ Natural, nonrigid self-discipline

⟠ A better perception of one's own vital needs

THEME: DISCIPLINE AND DOGMA

Key Symptoms

You're hard on yourself, have strict and rigid views, and suppress your vital needs for things such as food, sleep, and movement.

Recognize the spiritual misunderstanding . . .

Your unconscious wish is to achieve perfection and completeness. You are convinced that you know with absolute, theoretical precision how this can be accomplished. You keep strict discipline, hold fast to dogmatic theories and rules, and therefore misguidedly strive against the impulses of your Inner Guidance. You try to force the desired outcome, suppressing many of your natural needs.

... And correct it.

What is important now is to recognize that theories and rules are only guiding lights to help us develop our own goal-oriented strategies while taking into account our individual predispositions and needs. Not everything is for everyone.

When you continually feel that you have to force things, your Inner Guidance is showing you that something is going wrong. Once you identify your true needs and intentions, and use them as a basis for your actions, the results you are aiming for will be achieved much more easily and effortlessly.

Empowering statements:

❖ I pamper myself.
❖ I am flexible.
❖ I am spontaneous.

28. Scleranthus

The Balance Flower

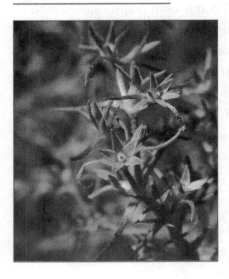

Promotes:

❀ Balanced mood

❀ Power to make decisions

❀ Consistent behavior

THEME:
FEELING PULLED IN OPPOSITE DIRECTIONS

Key Symptoms

One is indecisive, erratic, and inwardly unbalanced; opinions and moods change from one moment to the next.

Recognize the spiritual misunderstanding . . .

You have an unconscious desire to make decisions that will take into account all aspects of a situation in an appropriate way.

But because you identify completely with the predominant external conditions and do not listen to your own inner judgment, contact with your Inner Guidance is lost. You are always torn between two choices, one moment believing one is better, the next moment the other. The deciding itself becomes a bigger and bigger problem and can drag on interminably; only after a long struggle can you finally make a decision.

... And correct it.

It is important to seek your own balance, to orient yourself completely inward, to direct yourself toward your Inner Guidance. Only by these means will you receive the decision impulses that correspond to your own needs and support the unfolding of your Life Plan. As a result, you will have improved intuition, inner balance, and the ability to decide things quickly yet appropriately.

Empowering statements:

∽ I stand firm.
∽ I know what I want.
∽ I decide.

29. Star of Bethlehem
The Comfort Flower

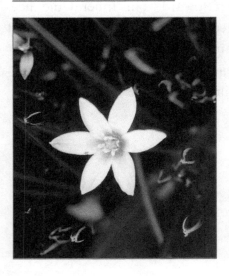

Promotes:

- ✃ The processing of unassimilated experiences

- ✃ The ability to react intuitively

THEME: TRAUMA

Key Symptoms

One has not yet overcome a mental or physical shock, which may have occurred long ago or more recently.

Recognize the spiritual misunderstanding . . .

You want to hold up your end in life, but when you become overwhelmed by a traumatic experience, you unconsciously decide not to let anything affect you anymore.

In order to avoid dealing with any more psychic injury, you shut off and construct a thick psychic shell. Everything is blocked: help from others and also, unfortunately, help from your Inner Guidance. This can be dangerous. This is why Star of Bethlehem is an ingredient in Rescue Remedy.

... And correct it.

It will be helpful to realize that any unexpected traumatic experience has the potential to mobilize the exact stores of energy that are needed in order to overcome the situation.

It will not be easy in the beginning; try to be aware of your unconscious shell and release it. Under the protection of your Inner Guidance, entrust yourself to the powerful energy game that is life. Only in this way can you become stronger psychically, absorb new experiences, and continue on your life's path.

Empowering statements:

  % I feel.
  % I breathe.
  % I am alive.

30. Sweet Chestnut

The Salvation Flower

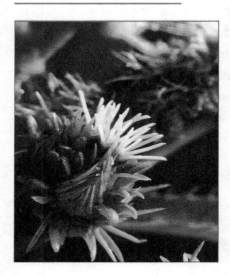

Promotes:

❧ Inner ability for psychic transformation

❧ Finding oneself

❧ Acceptance

❧ Trust in divine forces

THEME:
DESPERATION IN THE MIDST OF CRISIS

Key Symptoms

You believe you have reached the absolute limits of human suffering; utter hopelessness.

Recognize the spiritual misunderstanding . . .

When you are in deep despair, the following knowledge may not be exactly comforting, but still it will be very helpful for the future.

By wishing to master difficulties entirely on your own strength, you unconsciously have allowed an external or internal situation to come to an extreme point—because you have continually ignored the many small suggestions made by your Inner Guidance. Now the situation escalates. You are distressed and afraid of no longer being able to stand the pain; you expect to fall apart.

... And correct it.

Accept that there are moments in which you must give up all personal considerations and deliver yourself over completely to your Inner Guidance. Only then will new inspiration and ideas enter. Only then will new developments, waiting for so long, finally fall into place. Once again, you will see light at the end of the tunnel.

Empowering statements:

- ❀ I look out.
- ❀ I accept.
- ❀ I let it happen.

31. Vervain

The Enthusiasm Flower

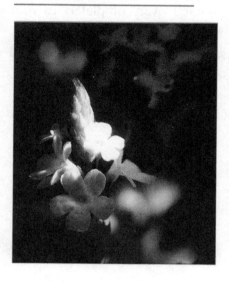

Promotes:

- S A proper sense of proportion

- S Constructive use of your own enthusiastic potential

- S A sense of the limits of tolerance in other people

THEME:
OVERZEALOUS AND OVERDONE

Key Symptoms

Your enthusiasm, even in support of a good cause, drains your energy; you become messianic, even fanatical.

Recognize the spiritual misunderstanding . . .

Your inner drive to contribute something constructive to the Greater Whole has caused you to get so carried away with an idea that you have lost your sense of proportion.

In your enthusiasm, you do not account for yourself, and without noticing it, you become increasingly distanced from your Inner Guidance. Due to this, you also lose sight of the personal limits of other people. You take things too far, leaving no space for argument. The initial open-mindedness of your conversation partners turns into resistance. You are thwarted.

... And correct it.

First, get back to your Inner Guidance! And leave some space. Get things back into balance. Accept that every person must follow his or her own concept of life.

The fact is that many roads lead to Rome. You can keep discussing things with many different people—but without putting pressure on them. Then the discussion can be enriching for everyone.

Empowering statements:

> ❦ I let it go.
> ❦ I give space to others.
> ❦ I pace my energy.

32. Vine
The Authority Flower

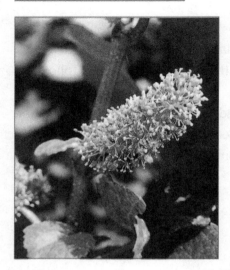

Promotes:

❗ Respect and empathy for fellow humans

❗ Tempering of excessive ambition to healthy ambition

❗ A constructive leadership style

THEME:
POWER AND AUTHORITY

Key Symptoms

There is a tendency to want to implement your own will at all costs; you have problems with power and authority.

Recognize the spiritual misunderstanding . . .

In your unconscious wish for a perfect unfolding of your Life Plan, you proceed in an excessively goal-oriented way, seeing only your own interests. People in whom this quality is strongly pronounced often had either too many or too few boundaries during childhood. Consequently, an appropriate relationship to the Greater Whole and to Inner Guidance has not been developed.

Since you inwardly believe that what you think is also right for other people, you fight tooth and nail to get your way. In doing this, you have no scruples, and even interfere in the Life Plans of others. Differing opinions and feelings do not reach you. For this reason, you are more feared than loved.

...And correct it.

Here, you must recognize and accept that you yourself are a part of the Greater Whole, and that your own Life Plan—like everyone else's—is also serving the greater good.

If you align your own interests with these higher interests, and consequently respect the needs of your fellow humans, you will no longer need to fight your way through. You will reach your goal automatically in the progression of a synergistic process. You will be voluntarily helped and gain the approval of others.

Empowering statements:
- ❧ I empathize.
- ❧ I show respect.
- ❧ I value and support.

34. Walnut
The Manifestation Flower

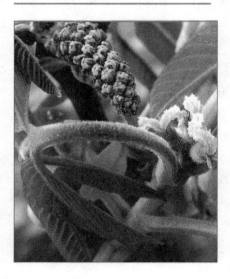

Promotes:

🕉 Protection from conventional thought patterns

🕉 Inner impartiality and independence

🕉 Inner stability

🕉 Strength of character

THEME: TOO EASILY INFLUENCED BY OTHERS

Key Symptoms

During new beginnings or times of change in your life, you may be too easily influenced, uncertain, and inconsistent.

Recognize the spiritual misunderstanding . . .

You find yourself in a phase of internal or external changes. You know exactly what the next step should be, but well-intentioned objections from others or worries about how your actions will affect others repeatedly hold you back from actually taking the planned step.

In this moment, your connection to your Inner Guidance is interrupted, and your development is on hold.

Perhaps the decision needs some time to mature so that enough inner resolve can develop for you to stand up to external resistance. But perhaps, due to outdated conventional principles, you have not yet left the old ways completely behind you.

... And correct it.

It is important to be clear on this fact: the unfolding of your Life Plan is always the first priority.

If you remain connected to your Inner Guidance, you will be able to tell whether and why you should hold back; or perhaps you will see what needs to be finalized before you can successfully start on your new phase.

Empowering statements:

- ❧ I am sure of myself.
- ❧ I stay true to myself.
- ❧ I go my own way.

34. Water Violet

The Communication Flower

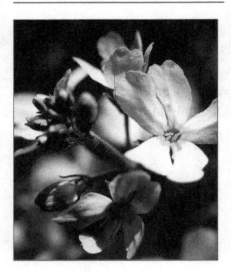

Promotes:

❒ Freedom from fear of intimacy

❒ The ability to approach other people

❒ Feelings of empathy

THEME: CLOSENESS AND DISTANCE

Key Symptoms

You are withdrawn, feel an inner distance from others, and may have an isolated feeling of superiority.

Recognize the spiritual misunderstanding . . .

In your unconscious effort to develop your individuality, you have learned, probably early in life, that no real help can be expected from other people. You erroneously believe that it is best to go it alone. For this reason, you are inclined to drop out of discussions quickly and to pull back from emotional situations.

This latent tendency to flee makes you emotionally isolated from your fellow humans and prevents the corresponding impulses from your Inner Guidance from coming through properly. You are internally self-sufficient. But because you allow very little input from others, your life becomes increasingly monotonous and insipid. Loneliness weighs down upon you.

... And correct it.

Here, the principle of unity provides food for thought: we are all part of the Greater Whole. Humans are not made for aloneness; we need each other in order to receive energetic prompts for our further developmental stages.

Once you fundamentally decide to allow more closeness in your life, your Inner Guidance will show you when it is time to open up and when it is time to draw back. In relaxed companionship, your life will become richer and stronger.

Empowering statements:

- ∾ I belong.
- ∾ I participate.
- ∾ I allow closeness.

35. White Chestnut
The Thought Flower

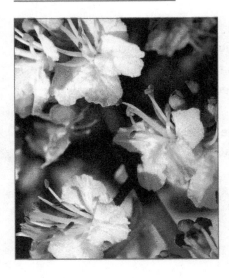

Promotes:

  ❀ Clarity of thought

  ❀ Mental focus

  ❀ Power of concentration

THEME: OVERACTIVE THOUGHTS

Key Symptoms

Certain thoughts—inner monologues and dialogues—circle persistently in your head, and you're unable to get rid of them.

Recognize the spiritual misunderstanding . . .

In your yearning for mental clarity and truth, you mistakenly seek to solve problems exclusively on the intellectual plane. Therefore, you are cut off from the universally ordering inspiration of your Inner Guidance.

    Feelings and needs that you do not perceive produce an increasing cyclical pressure in the whole energy system. This pressure also affects your mind and causes obsessive thoughts to run in accelerating circles. Since you are lacking the focus that is provided by conscious orientation toward your Inner Guidance, it's difficult to put your thought processes in order. You get more and more confused.

. . . And correct it.

It is important to become more conscious of the full spectrum of influences you perceive and to deliberately separate them from one another.

If, in doing this, you concentrate upon your Inner Guidance, all your thoughts will gradually be automatically structured in the direction of your Life Plan. Your thought energy will become more cohesive, and you will be able to use it constructively for the necessary processes of clarification.

Empowering statements:

    ❧ I feel the stillness.

    ❧ I feel clear.

    ❧ I guide my thoughts.

36. Wild Oat

The Vocational Calling Flower

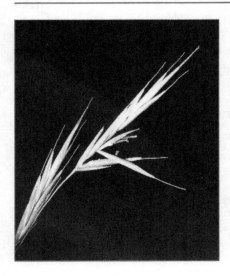

Promotes:

ॐ Clarity regarding one's goals

ॐ Orientation toward goals

ॐ Consistency

THEME:
INNER DISCONTENT, SEARCHING FOR A VISION

Key Symptoms

You are unclear about the direction you should follow. You are inwardly discontent because you cannot find your purpose in life.

Recognize the spiritual misunderstanding . . .

Like everyone, you are unconsciously aware of your uniqueness and want to express it. You want to be something special. Theoretically, all avenues of expression are open to you.

But if you mistakenly seek to realize this by looking only outward, you will not be oriented toward your Life Plan through your Inner Guidance. Your energies will be divided, and you will waste your time continually chasing new, enticing possibilities. Each time, the feeling will remain: you haven't yet found the "pot of gold." So you continue searching, going all over the place but never really feeling at home.

. . . And correct it.

Get ready for an about-face! Instead of looking for something special in the outside world, begin to connect, totally consciously, with your Inner Guidance.

Ask yourself: What is special about me? What are my unique qualities with which I can contribute to the Greater Whole?

From the wealth of possibilities, the really appropriate ones will emerge. Your true calling will become ever clearer. Your inner contentment will grow.

❦

Empowering statements:

Ω I see the meaning.
Ω I pursue my goal.
Ω I am fulfilled.

37. Wild Rose

The Zest for Life Flower

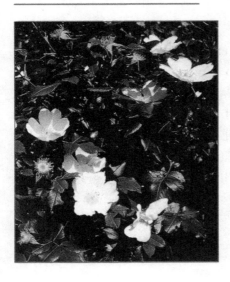

Promotes:

❧ Psychic activity

❧ New motivation for life

❧ Enjoyment of life

THEME: INTERNAL APATHY

Key Symptoms

Inwardly, you have given in; you are apathetic.

Recognize the spiritual misunderstanding . . .

You have an unconscious yearning to dive deeply into life. Possibly, during the first few days of life you were not sufficiently acknowledged or welcomed (for example, if you were born during some kind of intense crisis).

You therefore have the impression of not really existing. In this erroneous belief, you have not made contact with your Inner Guidance and have not demanded your share of cosmic life energy. Your original wish to surrender to life has fallen by the wayside. Instead, you surrender yourself apathetically to bad circumstances in life, and accept them as if they were par for the course. Other people cannot understand your apathy.

... And correct it.

It is high time to recognize that nothing is final in this life. New life can always rise up from the ruins.

Every moment is a new opportunity to resume contact with your Inner Guidance and to participate actively in the great game of life.

Your Life Plan still offers countless new and exciting opportunities!

Empowering statements:

    🙞 I want to live.
    🙞 I demand life.
    🙞 I seize my chance.

38. Willow

The Destiny Flower

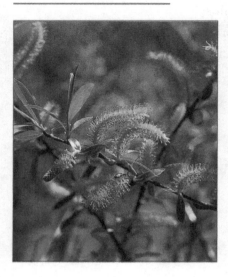

Promotes:

₧ Responsibility for oneself

₧ A constructive attitude toward life

₧ Creativity in one's tasks

THEME:
BITTERNESS AND RESENTMENT

Key Symptoms

You feel yourself to be at the mercy of circumstances. You are embittered and see yourself as a victim of fate.

Recognize the spiritual misunderstanding . . .

In the unconscious, childlike yearning for a paradise in which all wishes are fulfilled, you confuse the realm of wishes with the realm of reality.

This condition often originates from the phase of childhood development in which one experiences the world as a powerless infant, not yet realizing that one can cause or influence events.

In your adult life, when fate does not bring what you hoped for, you resent it and bitterly draw away from your Inner Guidance. If something unwelcome happens, you search automatically for the cause in the outside world; you are unable to see your own part in it. This leads to negative moods and causes your life's path to deviate.

...And correct it.

Stop sulking! Take responsibility and recognize that in the ups and downs of life there are always causes *and* effects, giving *and* taking, action *and* reaction. Accept your Inner Guidance and practice, with its help, ways in which you can constructively influence situations and your fellow humans. There are undreamed-of possibilities! Your perception of life will become positive, and more and more of your wishes will come true.

Empowering statements:

- ❀ I am powerful.
- ❀ I have authority.
- ❀ I take responsibility.

39. Rescue Remedy

The Emergency Remedy

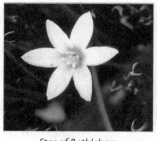

Star of Bethlehem

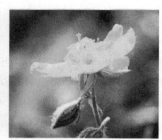

Rock Rose

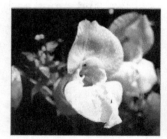

Impatiens

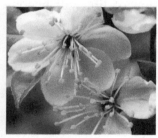

Cherry Plum

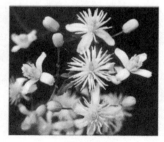

Clematis

Rescue Remedy is the best-known and most widely used of all the Bach Flower Essences. In 1930 Bach saved a fisherman's life with it. Since then, Rescue Remedy has given countless people immediate, palpable calm and reassurance in the face of emergencies or stressful situations and has often saved their lives indirectly.

Rescue Remedy works for every personality type. With this

combination of flowers, Bach pinpointed an overarching archetypal pattern of human reactions: the process that every person undergoes when an event is so overwhelming that the integration of Soul, spirit, and body becomes endangered.

In this sense, Bach was ahead of his time and anticipated the findings of modern stress research. He identified the following five behavior patterns in reactions to extraordinary situations.

Star of Bethlehem	Fear and shock: the trauma reflex
Rock Rose	Feelings of terror and panic; nervous overreaction
Impatiens	Mental stress and tension, excessive impulses to act
Cherry Plum	Fear of losing control
Clematis	The tendency to give in; the feeling of being far away, often taking place before loss of consciousness

Rescue Remedy affords emotional stabilization and relaxation of body and Soul, consequently creating the best conditions for any physical treatment that might be needed. However, Rescue Remedy is not a substitute for emergency medical treatment.

Rescue Remedy is not a substitute for Bach Flower Therapy, either. At best it is an initial step to be taken prior to therapy, a kind of psychic bandage.

Rescue Remedy can be taken in combination with individual Flower Therapy and can be taken repeatedly and intermittently.

DOSAGE FOR RESCUE REMEDY

Four drops in a glass of water, sipped at intervals; repeat as needed.

RESCUE CREAM

For minor bodily injury such as burns, sprains, cuts, and sudden skin irritation, Rescue Cream is recommended as a salve. The cream contains essences of the five Rescue Flowers, as well as Crab Apple, the Cleansing Flower.

WHEN SHOULD
ONE TAKE RESCUE REMEDY?

When one is psychically upset, for example:

- ※ After a family argument
- ※ After receiving disappointing news

Prior to an uncomfortable experience, for example:

- ※ Surgery
- ※ A court date

When one has received a shock, for example:

- ※ After a traffic accident
- ※ After a household accident
- ※ Following a heart attack

When one is obliged to work in a stressful atmosphere, for example:

- ※ Surrounded by a large group of people
- ※ Under great time pressure

A Note
for Practitioners

Are there more crisis situations today than there used to be? Looking around, one might believe this to be the case. One might also have the impression that today, as we face an increasing number of new and difficult challenges, our present strategies are becoming less and less reliable.

Often enough in these times, the experience gained by older generations is no longer applicable. Higher values, and societal and moral paradigms such as family, school, and church, are now rarely viewed as helpful for finding direction. What the future holds is hard to guess, given the fast-paced tempo of today's continually changing society. It seems almost impossible to make any long-term plans for our lives.

What remains for individuals, what is becoming ever more important for them—even when they have no reliable role models in life—is the path of individual crisis management, based on a few specific insights and perceptions. These insights and perceptions can ultimately be attained only with the aid of a good connection to one's own Inner Guidance. For many people, this is too much to ask, because they have neither learned nor practiced competent self-management in crisis situations. This is the task at hand!

In these circumstances, the concept of the original Bach Flower Therapy is even more relevant today than when it first appeared more than seventy years ago. Its persuasive success originated in an ingenious idea—a therapeutic connection between two important levels of human existence.

≈ On the spiritual level, the precise pattern of the thirty-eight psychic potentials of human nature provides ideal orientation and guidance.

≈ On the material level, the self-chosen combination of Bach Flowers gives the seeker a means for receiving palpable help and support in crisis situations. Consequently, it becomes easier to deal responsibly with crisis situations and use them as opportunities for growth.

From a contemporary viewpoint, Bach Flower Therapy is a perfect example of the famous principle of salutogenesis, a term coined by medical sociologist Aaron Antonovsky. Salutogenesis describes the relationship between health and illness as a continuous variable—the "health-ease vs. dis-ease continuum." Antonovsky noted that some people became ill in response to stress while others manage to develop a positive attitude that helps them cope and maintain their equilibrium.

As developed by Dr. Edward Bach, this concept offers two further advantages for building competence for crisis management.

1. In crisis situations, one may get lost in guilt and self-reproach and may never even get beyond the level of personal shock. By perceiving and correcting "spiritual misunderstandings," Bach Flower principles make it possible to move into the level of the observer right from the start.

It is possible to recognize one's own behavior in the context of precisely defined reaction patterns and to correct these reactions, at least theoretically. This allows one to gain distance and—

supported by the energy of the ingested Flower Essences—to take first definite steps in a new direction.

2. This makes Bach Flower Therapy the ideal complement and supplement to all therapy concepts based on detoxification, purification, or rehabilitation—whether in mainstream medicine, psychology, or physical therapy.

Because the effect of Bach Flowers does not take place on the physical level, it combines well with all other forms of therapy. There are no interactions. On the contrary, as an accompaniment to other types of therapy, Bach Flower Therapy has been shown to be highly effective.

About the Author

Mechthild Scheffer, an international specialist and pioneer in the original Bach Flower Therapy, translated the work of Dr. Edward Bach into German in 1981. Since then, she has built systematically upon the original Bach Flower Therapy and made groundbreaking contributions to its development.

For decades, Mechthild Scheffer served as a representative of the English Bach Center in Germany, Austria, and Switzerland. During more than thirty years of practice and research, she has published many articles and thirteen books; some of these are fundamental to the original Bach Flower Therapy and have been translated into several languages.

Mechthild Scheffer founded the *Institute für Bach-Blütentherapie, Forschung und Lehre* in Hamburg, Vienna, and Zürich. Her instructive seminars have been attended by thousands of clients and therapists. Currently, Mechthild Scheffer is involved in integrating the original Bach Flower Therapy into an expanded concept of salutogenesis and in initiatives to provide for future psychosocial well-being.

Help in the selection and exploration of crisis situations was provided by Dieter Brandt, Dagmar Gehm, Ingrid Haring, Mag. Claudia Killermann, Dr. Max Segeth, Dr. Eva Tröbinger, and Beate Wüpper. Thank you for your support and collaboration in the writing of this book.

Thanks also to the participants in our seminars, and our clients for their contributions and engagement in discussions and conversations. The assistance of the extended Bach Flower community has also been invaluable.

BOOKS OF RELATED INTEREST

Bach Flower Therapy
Theory and Practice
by Mechthild Scheffer

The Encyclopedia of Bach Flower Therapy
by Mechthild Scheffer

Mastering Bach Flower Therapies
A Guide to Diagnosis and Treatment
by Mechthild Scheffer

Advanced Bach Flower Therapy
A Scientific Approach to Diagnosis and Treatment
by Götz Blome, M.D.

Bach Flower Remedies for Children
A Parents' Guide
by Barbara Mazzarella

New Bach Flower Body Maps
Treatment by Topical Application
by Dietmar Krämer

New Bach Flower Therapies
Healing the Emotional and Spiritual Causes of Illness
by Dietmar Krämer

Bach Flower Remedies to the Rescue
by Gregory Vlamis

INNER TRADITIONS • BEAR & COMPANY
P.O. Box 388
Rochester, VT 05767
1-800-246-8648
www.InnerTraditions.com

Or contact your local bookseller

☐ I feel as though I've failed as a dog owner.   *Larch*

☐ My great ambition is to train my dog without
   anyone else's help.   *Vine*

☐ I don't like the idea that trainers would have
   more influence over my dog than I do.   *Chicory, Holly, Vine*

☐ It makes me angry that my dog doesn't obey me.
   Sometimes I even hate him.   *Holly*

Vine

Centaury

Cerato

Larch

Chicory

Holly